Praise for *Feeling Stressed Is Optional*

"*Feeling Stressed Is Optional* offers an essential lifeline to physicians grappling with the all-too-common struggles of chronic stress and burnout. As a chief wellness officer, I find Robyn's holistic approach, grounded in Lifestyle Medicine, to be both profoundly empathetic and remarkably practical. This book is an invaluable guide for any healthcare professional seeking to survive and truly thrive in their personal and professional life."

—**Amber Orman, MD, DipABLM, Chief Wellness Officer, AdventHealth Medical Group**

"*Feeling Stressed Is Optional* by Dr. Robyn Tiger is an invaluable resource for anyone seeking practical, evidence-based strategies to manage stress effectively. Dr. Tiger expertly integrates the pillars of Lifestyle Medicine with experiential activities that empower readers to take control of their well-being. This book is a must-read for cultivating resilience and leading a more balanced life."

—**Melissa Sundermann, DO, FACOI, DipABLM, FACLM, Lifestyle Medicine physician**

"*Feeling Stressed Is Optional* is the best place to begin if you are looking for achievable, small goals to improve your lifestyle. As a leader in physician well-being for over a decade, Robyn Tiger's book is long overdue and a gift to our world. This is an excellent resource for physicians to establish camaraderie like in the good old days of the doctors' lounge!

—**Michelle L. Thompson, DO, AOBFP, ABOIM, DipABLM, FACLM, Medical Director Lifestyle Medicine, University of Pittsburgh Medical Center**

"Dr. Tiger did an amazing job of combining her lived experiences and clinical expertise to distill down the science and art of stress management in our daily lives. While frequently underappreciated, both acute and chronic stress are mediators of many common diseases. This book uses a unique approach by tapping into the power of the pillars of Lifestyle Medicine to mitigate stress. I strongly endorse this book as a Lifestyle Medicine expert and an interventional cardiologist dealing with high-stress situations daily."

—Koushik R. Reddy, MD, FACC, FACLM, DipABLM, LMI, Lifestyle Medicine physician

"As a physician who is deeply committed to lifestyle and integrative medicine, I am profoundly impressed by Dr. Robyn Tiger's book, *Feeling Stressed Is Optional*. Dr. Tiger masterfully combines her extensive medical expertise with practical, evidence-based strategies to offer a comprehensive guide for managing stress. This book empowers individuals to take control of their well-being. Dr. Tiger's compassionate and insightful guidance makes complex concepts accessible and actionable, providing invaluable tools for both personal and professional growth."

—Dawn M. Mussallem, DO, DipABLM, Medical Director Humanities in Medicine, Chair Employee Well-Being Mayo Clinic Florida, Assistant Professor of Medicine, Jacoby Center for Breast Health, Mayo Clinic Cancer Center

"When I first met Dr. Robyn Tiger at a Lifestyle Medicine conference in 2022, I was in awe (and admittedly) a bit jealous of how calm, cool, and collected she was. How did she "have it all together"? Robyn's heartfelt words are relatable, genuine, and full of passion. Her message resonates not only with physicians but with anyone who struggles with feelings of imposter syndrome and burnout."

—Christina Lucas Vougiouklakis, DO, DipABLM, FACLM, Clinic Medical Director/Director of Lifestyle Medicine and Osteopathic Medicine, ProMedica

"*Feeling Stressed Is Optional* is a transformative guide that I am incredibly grateful to have as a resource. As a busy physician, I truly appreciate how Dr. Tiger masterfully integrates tools from Lifestyle Medicine into a "stress-free toolbox." Her approach is both practical and empowering. I know this book will help many on their journey to a healthier, more balanced life."

—Amy Comander, MD, DipABLM, Director of Lifestyle Medicine, Mass General Cancer Center, Director of Breast Oncology and Survivorship, Mass General Cancer Center at Massachusetts General Hospital in Waltham and at Newton-Wellesley Hospital

"Physician burnout has risen as high as 62.8% in 2021. Having experienced burnout, dissatisfaction, and depression myself, the first three steps for a "way out" are awareness, vulnerability, and courage. It is time to be more of a *human being* than just a *human doing*. Physicians are people, too, and we have a responsibility to ourselves and a duty to the people we serve to put *the oxygen mask on ourselves first!* Dr. Robyn's book lays it out in a simple, concise approach to applying her strategies. You'll be glad you did."

—Colin Zhu, DO, FACLM, DipABLM, chef, author of *Thrive Medicine: How to Cultivate Your Desires and Elevate Your Life*, founder of TheChefDoc, host of the *Thrive Bites* podcast

"Dr. Robyn Tiger has created an indispensable master class in self-care for all of us, but especially for those in the healing professions. Through quotes, anecdotes, experiential learning, and a perfect blend of scientific evidence mixed with best-friend conversational style, Robyn guides us to examine our current levels of stress and dis-ease and then challenges us to take concrete action—shifting the paradigm toward thriving instead of just surviving. You will want to share it with everyone you love!"

—Meagan L. Grega, MD, FACLM, DipABLM, DipABFM, Co-Founder and Chief Medical Officer, Kellyn Foundation

FEELING STRESSED IS
Optional

Transforming the Life of the Chronically Stressed Physician

ROBYN TIGER, MD, DipABLM
THE SELF-CARE DOCTOR

Feeling Stressed Is Optional
Transforming the Life of the Chronically Stressed Physician
Robyn Tiger © 2024

The author and Aloha Publishing support copyright and the sharing of thoughts and ideas it enables. Thank you for buying an authorized edition of this book and honoring our request to obtain permission for any use of any part of this publication, whether reproduced, transmitted in any form or by any means, electronic, mechanical, photocopying, recording, or otherwise, or stored in a retrieval system. Your honorable actions support all writers and allow the publishing industry to continue publishing books for all readers. All rights reserved.

While the publisher and author have used their best efforts in preparing this book, they make no representations or warranties with respect to the accuracy or completeness of this book and specifically disclaim any implied warranties of merchantability or fitness for a particular purpose. No warranty may be created or extended by sales representatives or written sales materials. The stories and interviews in this book are true although the names and identifiable information may have been changed to maintain confidentiality.

The publisher and author shall have neither liability nor responsibility to any person or entity with respect to loss of profit or property, damage, or injury caused or alleged to be caused directly or indirectly by the information contained in this book. The information presented herein is in no way intended as a substitute for counseling or other professional guidance.

Hardcover ISBN: 978-1-61206-324-9
Softcover ISBN: 978-1-61206-325-6
eBook ISBN: 978-1-61206-326-3

To purchase this book at quantity discounts, contact Aloha Publishing at alohapublishing@gmail.com or StressFreeMD.net

Published by:

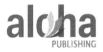

In partnership with Stress Free LLC

Printed in the United States of America

Contents

Foreword	11
Introduction	17
How to Use This Book	31
Chapter 1: Pillars of Lifestyle Medicine	45
Chapter 2: Stress Less, Relax Better	53
Chapter 3: Stress Less, Eat Better	81
Chapter 4: Stress Less, Sleep Better	109
Chapter 5: Stress Less, Move Better	137
Chapter 6: Stress Less, Connect Better	161
Chapter 7: Stress Less, Say "No" Better	183
Chapter 8: Stress Less, Thrive Better	205
Hungry for More?	211
About the Author	215
Resources	217
Links	219
Acknowledgments	223
Book Club Questions	227
Podcast and Media Questions	231
Citations	233

Dedication

To my three physician friends who died from suicide and live on through these teachings.

And to all physicians and physicians in training who deserve and are in need of stress prevention and relief to come back home to their true selves and live their happiest, healthiest, and most fulfilling lives.

Foreword

As a stressed-out, anxious, and depressed cardiologist on the front lines of care, I spent years trying to heal the hearts of others without truly listening to or caring for my own. I found myself caught in a cycle of burnout, disengaged from the very work that once inspired me. Like so many of my colleagues, I was driven into medicine by a deep desire to care for others and make the world a better place. But over time, the countless organizational and systemic factors that dominate our profession began to wear me down, disconnecting me from my purpose and leaving me feeling isolated and overwhelmed.

The crisis of burnout among physicians is real and pervasive. We are often expected to function at the highest levels, juggling the demands of patient care, administrative duties, and personal responsibilities, all while keeping our own struggles hidden. I wish I had Robyn's book when I was hiding my own pain and shame from my colleagues, feeling like I had nowhere to turn. This book would have been the lifeline I needed—a guide not only to surviving but thriving in a career that often seems to take more than it gives.

Robyn's journey, as shared in this book, is nothing short of inspirational. She courageously opens up about her own struggles with chronic stress and burnout, a story that resonates deeply. Her experience is a powerful reminder that even those who seem to have it all together can be silently suffering. The case presentation at the beginning of chapter 1 paints a vivid picture of a life unraveling due to the cumulative toll of stress—a life that could easily belong to any one of us.

Through her personal transformation, Robyn discovered the life-saving impact of self-care and holistic health practices. She uses lessons learned from her own journey to create a comprehensive, actionable guide designed to help others find their way out of the darkness of stress and burnout. The chapters that follow are structured around the essential pillars of Lifestyle Medicine, offering practical strategies for stress management, nutrition, sleep, physical activity, social connections, and more.

As I read this book, it felt like having my own master coach by my side, available whenever I needed guidance. Robyn's writing is so approachable and clear; it's as if she is sitting right here with me, having a warm conversation. The instructions are practical and easy to follow, making this an all-in-one guide for busy doctors who have given so much to others and paid the price with their health and well-being.

What sets this book apart is the palpable empathy, compassion, and love that Robyn pours into her insights and instructions. The book's holistic approach addresses the most common ways we become chronically stressed, helps us reverse them, and provides specific, tested tools to create the life we've always dreamed of, rather than merely avoiding pain. It's impossible to read this book and come away unchanged.

I've had the privilege to know Robyn and experience her guidance firsthand, through her teachings in yoga, meditation, stress reduction, and coaching. I've also had the honor of leading a weekend mountain retreat with her, focused on physician well-being, where I witnessed the profound impact she has on others. Robyn's ability to connect deeply with people and change lives is truly remarkable.

This book will serve as a resource for me to return to again and again and also to share with my colleagues and patients. Lifestyle Medicine can often be complicated, but Robyn has a way of clearly communicating the essence of each pillar, including the why and the how. Most importantly, she helps us understand the science of habit change and how to do the hard work of implementing change in our own lives and helping others.

As you read this book, I encourage you to embrace the tools and techniques Robyn shares. Whether it's adopting a new dietary habit, incorporating mindfulness practices into your day, or finding ways to connect more deeply with loved ones, each small change can have a significant impact on your health and happiness. The journey to wellness is a personal one, but with Robyn's guidance, you don't have to walk it alone.

In closing, I want to express my deep gratitude to Robyn for her courage and dedication in writing this book. Her work is a testament to the power of self-care and the resilience of the human spirit. As you turn the pages, may you find the inspiration, motivation, and tools to create a healthier, more fulfilling life for yourself and those you love.

Warmly,

Dr. Jonathan Fisher,
Cardiologist, mindfulness teacher, and organizational well-being leader; co-founder, Ending Clinician Burnout Global Community; author of *Just One Heart: A Cardiologist's Guide to Healing, Health, and Happiness*

Welcome!

Follow the QR code below to watch a short welcome video:

Introduction

"Do not go where the path may lead. Go instead where there is no path and leave a trail."

—Ralph Waldo Emerson

Do you want to hear about an interesting case? Let's start off by exploring it together:

CASE PRESENTATION

Chief Complaint: "I'm falling apart, have hit rock bottom, and fear for my life."

History of Present Illness: A 42-year-old female physician presents with a several-year history of multiple progressive complaints. Migraine headaches began in her early 30s during residency training, accompanied by intense vomiting and intolerance for light and sound. Additionally, patient describes intermittent paresthesias with numbness and tingling in her hands and feet, causing temporary loss of function. She is particularly frightened by this symptom. She mentions this has occurred on multiple occasions including losing sensation in her hands when holding biopsy guns while performing breast biopsies, holding the steering wheel of a car, and holding knives when cutting vegetables. The patient describes painful tension throughout her whole body, which has resulted in significant decreased range of motion. Additional symptoms include spontaneously bleeding gums, tinnitus, vertigo, abdominal pain following eating with distention, poor bowel habits alternating between constipation and diarrhea, and gastroesophageal reflux with burning chest pain. Her fear of a debilitating neurological disease combined with her other symptoms have caused extensive sleep disruption and lack of focus and concentration throughout the day. Emotionally she suffers from anxiety and excessive worry, is very reactive, and admits to suicidal ideation. Patient has lost three physician colleagues to suicide, which exacerbates this situation.

Allergies: No known medicine or food allergies. Severe latex allergy.

Social History: Patient is an actively practicing female diagnostic radiologist, happily married with two young, healthy children. She volunteers for multiple community organizations and at her children's school. She follows a vegan diet and exercises daily, running and training for races.

Past Medical History: Mild hypercholesterolemia

Past Surgical History: Left knee arthroscopy during childhood

Medications: Crestor 5 mg/day

Review of Systems: No additional findings

Physical Examination: Within normal limits

Workup Included:

- **Specialist consults**: Neurologist, gastroenterologist, psychologist, periodontist

- **Imaging**: Negative MRI of spine, negative MRI of hips
- **Labs**: All within normal limits
- **Medications**: Medications for gastroesophageal reflux, muscular tension, migraine headaches, neuropathy, mood elevation
- **Therapy**: Physical therapy, acupuncture, massage, chiropractic, mental health

Patient's symptoms persisted on medications and therapy with no relief. The medications made her feel worse overall so she stopped taking them.

A CHANGE IN PERSPECTIVE

What were this patient's next steps? She desperately wanted to relieve her symptoms and get back to "normal" again. Western medicine didn't seem to have the answer. She began to envision the journey of her life as a fork in the road splitting into two paths: the path that three of her friends she'd lost to suicide had taken, or a new path.

Fearing for her life, she decided to think outside the box to find a different way to resolve all of her symptoms. And guess what? She actually did! Every single symptom resolved completely, with no medications and no therapy. *Amazing*, right?

Guess what again? The patient was *me*!

You may be thinking, "No way! Really?" Well yes, *really!*

I was the only physician to make my correct diagnosis: *chronic stress.*

I was the only physician to prescribe my correct Rx: *self-care.*

And I have spent over a decade sharing what I learned, *what we were never taught in medical training and deserve to know*! And this is why we are here together so I can share what I learned with you, too.

While my symptoms were severe (and terrifying at times), many of the things I experienced are unfortunately common among physicians who suffer from chronic stress. Let me ask you this: Do you see yourself in any of these symptoms? One? More than one? If the answer is yes, know that you are not alone.

Luckily my story ends differently than the stories of many other physicians—I found a way out, a way to relieve my stress and the accompanying symptoms. With my newfound tools, I built an incredibly happy and healthy life for myself, and I am here to show you how you can too!

This personal transformation led me to pivot and dedicate my career to passionately helping others do the same.

A DEEPER DIVE INTO MY JOURNEY

My life looked perfect from the outside: I was happily married to another physician, had two amazing little kids, and had a beautiful home. But little by little, I developed all of these seemingly disconnected symptoms that interfered with my daily life. I was constantly in pain: physical, emotional, psychological, and spiritual—down to my very soul.

Like most physicians, I'd been taught that caring for myself came second to caring for my patients and family, and that lesson was reinforced throughout my training and medical practice.

When my situation began to feel hopeless, I started to have a lot of dark, scary thoughts like "I can't spend another day like this." I

INTRODUCTION

didn't want to be here anymore—life was too painful. Every day I'd have to wake up and go through more pain. Some days I was commuting three to four hours and was trying to be a good mother to a toddler and a baby. I had no social life because there was no time for socializing. It felt like the movie *Groundhog Day*, where every day was the same. However, there was no happy ending in sight.

All of this suffering added up to a lot of guilt and shame. Who was I to complain? I had a stable job, a wonderful family, a dog, a beautiful house, and nice cars. It looked like I was living the American dream. Despite how wonderful my life appeared on the outside, I felt like I was dying on the inside. I didn't feel present to appreciate all that I had.

My baby would smile at me and I would see it, but I wouldn't feel it. I began making several dumb mistakes, leading to further guilt and stress. I forgot my son's nebulizer when we went on vacation and I spent hours on the phone with the pediatrician and the hotel to get his medications and a nebulizer rental. Another time, we attended a show and I saw people sitting in our seats, so I asked the usher for assistance. Apparently our tickets were for the day prior. My kids complained the whole time that they couldn't see or hear as the only remaining seats were in the "nosebleed" section. Once I brought our family to the wrong airline terminal on Christmas Day (even though I had typed in the correct flight information to send to the family the night before). It was an absolute circus to get all of us and our many pieces of luggage to the correct terminal among the droves of people. And there are more and more examples. With each mistake, I felt worse and worse about myself.

As I grew more desperate for solutions, my treatments and appointments grew to an overwhelming level. Each specialist focused on a different symptom and gave me a pill—"a pill for an ill." But nobody looked for the actual *root cause* of all the symptoms, the "why" behind everything I was experiencing.

Amidst all of this, I was losing physician friends and colleagues who were dying from suicide. I was suffering from suicidal thoughts of my own. And the medical field was drastically changing, so we were all being asked to do more and more work in the same amount of time. Moral injury had strongly set in. It was not the job I had signed up for, and my intense disappointment was dampening the spark that had driven me to go into medicine in the first place.

MY PIVOT

Eventually, I began seeing a therapist. After a few sessions, she said, "You know, you're really #$%& amazing! Do you not realize this? Can you see yourself through my eyes?"

The therapist went on to tell me I could keep coming if I wanted, but she didn't think she could do anything else for me. So I wondered what I could do next. I thought, *What does she see that she thinks is amazing? How can I look at things differently?*

It sounds simple, but that one interaction caused a significant switch in my perspective. I realized that I was taking a pile of pills every day, which only made me feel worse. I was inundated with different therapies and experiencing further stress as I tried to make it to all of my appointments. I was eating what I considered a healthy diet. And I was also a gym rat, exercising daily (sometimes more than once a day) at the gym, pushing myself hard because it helped me feel more present in my body and temporarily drew my attention away from my intrusive thoughts.

INTRODUCTION

As I drove home from therapy that day, I realized I was out of ideas. I thought, *This isn't working. I don't want to take these pills anymore. What else am I supposed to do? There isn't another specialist I can think of seeing. There's not another imaging test I can think of getting. There's not another blood test that would make sense.*

I feared if I didn't find a solution I would end up like my physician friends who had died from suicide.

I decided that was not an option.

Around that time, I'd been seeing an advertisement in the local papers for a Yoga 101 series at a studio down the road from my home. I did a lot of eye-rolling because I thought yoga was just a bunch of people wearing colorful spandex, listening to weird music, twisting their bodies into painful upside-down positions, and chanting strange words. (If you think this too, you are not alone.) But I was at rock bottom. *Why not give it a try?* I thought. If not for me, I'd try it at least to make a change for my kids and my husband, so I hesitantly signed up for the series.

FROM EYE-ROLLING TO EYES OPEN

I remember that day like it was yesterday. The first class of the series started on a weeknight at 7:30, and I could barely keep my eyes open because I was exhausted after working a full day, reading tons of imaging studies, performing many procedures, driving home, feeding and bathing my kids, handing them off to my husband, and then running out the door to make it on time to class.

I remember walking into the studio head down, anxious, stressed, and exhausted, not making eye contact, questioning my decision, and thinking, *I am just wasting my time. This is stupid. There is so much work I could be doing at home.*

However, 60 minutes later when the class ended, I felt like I'd done a 180: awake yet calm, grounded, and clear—and my body didn't hurt for the first time in years. (Yes, I said *awake,* even though I'd completely dragged myself in.)

This yoga series was very informal, allowing for questions and answers along the way, and the instructor was a professor at a local university. She was authentic and intelligent, and she explained things in a scientific way. She shared techniques for breathing and movement and the effects those have on our bodies and minds. Over those five weeks, I felt so much better physically, mentally, emotionally, psychologically, and spiritually. The way she presented lessons allowed my intellectual brain to engage. It prompted me to dive into medical literature and learn the physiology behind the shift I was experiencing.

What was my main takeaway?

> **I realized that I was learning how to dial down the chronic stress response that had been wreaking havoc on my whole self.**

Over the next few weeks, as I began to implement more tools into my daily routine, all of my symptoms began to fade away. I was calmer and sleeping better. Within a few months, I didn't notice any of the major symptoms anymore—I was getting better and better. Eventually, every single symptom went away, even the most worrisome symptoms, including the paresthesias and even the suicidal ideation.

INTRODUCTION

It wasn't a pill that helped me. It wasn't therapy. I came to understand that what cured me was decreasing the chronic stress hormone, cortisol, and decreasing the elevated cytokine levels from inflammation in my body that had been causing all of my symptoms.

I no longer had to talk myself out of bed every morning. I now knew how to make myself feel better. I realized that these changes were not only positively affecting me, but others in my life were noticing a new me as well. People loved being around me again! My staff, friends, and family all noticed and wanted to know the secret sauce. I frequently heard, "I want what she's having!"

One of the most eye-opening statements came from my daughter, who was very young at the time. We were having a conversation where I was actively listening and asking her questions when she paused, looked me straight in the eyes, and said, "Mommy, I really love it when you look at me when I'm talking to you, Mommy." (She used to put my name as bookends on her sentences.) With that statement, I lost my breath. Her words made me realize I hadn't been present for her, and probably for so many others, for quite a long while. I held back the tears of both sadness at my lack of presence and gratitude for how my life had begun to change for the better for myself and others I care about.

THE PHYSICIAN AS A FOREVER STUDENT

As a physician and therefore a forever student, the rapid transformation I saw in my own health drove me to study what I was learning more deeply to satisfy my left brain's curiosity. I became certified as a yoga teacher through a 200-hour training, never thinking I would teach anyone else, but simply because I wanted to educate myself. It was there that I learned about the field of yoga therapy, applying the principles of yoga at a higher level to help others with a myriad of symptoms of illnesses and diseases. Hearing about this made my ears perk up! I was immediately drawn to this method of "doctoring in a different way." I was so inspired I decided to complete the three-year 1000-hour yoga therapy certification.

During that training, I experienced continued improvement of my symptoms as well as the profound healing effects of iRest® meditation, originally developed for Walter Reed Army Hospital to help our military relieve the suffering from PTSD. iRest® meditation has also been found to relieve chronic pain and is as effective as pain medication because pain outside of trauma or illness is most commonly due to stress. The Department of Defense has declared iRest® meditation a Tier 1 treatment for chronic pain for this very reason. This meditation taught me how to be with and *process* life's experiences, which is unique compared to most other types of meditation.

After spending many years focused on utilizing body-based stress relief tools and teaching others how to do the same, I found another set of helpful tools that focused on the mind. I learned how to work with my thoughts through a cognitive behavior therapy-based life coaching program. As a lifelong learner, what did I then do? I went on to become a certified life coach! Adding these mindset skills to my body-based skills was an important piece of the puzzle for effective healing and growth.

But that's not all! I then learned about a *whole new way* to approach medicine. I found a place where I could apply all that I had already learned and *so much more*. I knew I'd found my new home: *Lifestyle Medicine*.

INTRODUCTION

DISCOVERING LIFESTYLE MEDICINE

After experiencing this incredible transformation in my own life, I was strongly drawn to support my physician colleagues and help the healthcare community through what I'd learned. To start, I connected with my local medical society, the Western Carolina Medical Society. I met with their CEO, Miriam Schwarz, who welcomed me with open arms to become a partner in their Healthy Healer Program, a nonprofit that supports their members, and I was invited to their annual event. It was there that I met a physician, Dr. Ginger Poulton, who was the founder of the Lifestyle Medicine Advancement Group. She was very interested in my initiatives and invited me to join this group as well as attend a meeting she was hosting at her home. I'd never heard of Lifestyle Medicine before, so I immediately went home and Googled it. My eyes opened wide upon finding the American College of Lifestyle Medicine and their life-changing approach to medicine.

That night I read about the six pillars of Lifestyle Medicine: nutrition, physical activity, restorative sleep, social connection, stress management, and avoidance of risky substances. They covered what I'd been learning, implementing myself, and teaching others. I was so excited—and I wondered, *Where have you been all my life?*

When I attended the meeting, I was surrounded by people just like me, people who understood my passion and were board-certified in this discipline and teaching these pillars to their patients. I was exhilarated—I'd finally found where I belonged.

After learning about my background, another physician at the meeting connected me with an education administrator at the American College of Lifestyle Medicine, and I was thrilled to learn that they were in need of content creation for the pillar of stress management. They warmly welcomed me to serve as lead faculty and subject matter expert in stress management to develop content for the new *Foundations of Lifestyle Medicine Board Review Manual* section titled "Emotional and Mental Health Assessment and Interventions." I was so excited about the opportunity to educate thousands of other healthcare professionals and their millions of patients in this way. I got goosebumps imagining the impact and ripple effect of my teachings. They also invited me to sit for the boards and, as a lifelong learner, I dove headfirst into my studies. I enjoyed it immensely and am proud to say that I am a board-certified Lifestyle Medicine physician, the field of medicine with which I feel most aligned and at home.

YOUR PATH TO STRESS PREVENTION AND RELIEF

If any part of my story has resonated with you, I want you to know that you're not alone. Your story may look similar to mine or it may be different, but no matter where you are or what you're experiencing, know you *can* improve your relationship with stress.

Although I was drawn to write this book to support my colleagues in the medical profession, anyone dealing with chronic stress can benefit from the teachings and techniques found in these pages. I have written in a way that everyone can understand.

I am particularly passionate about helping physicians both prevent and relieve stress and burnout. The physician suicide rate, pre-pandemic, was twice the national average and is expected to continue to rise. The most recent Medscape statistics report that 60% of physicians don't even take care of their own health.[1]

INTRODUCTION

How can physicians be the gatekeepers of health when they themselves are not well?

Chronic stress is America's number one health problem, and 70-90% of all visits to primary care physicians are for stress-related problems.[2] Remember physicians are patients too, with job stress being the leading cause of stress. In order to most effectively address it, we need to start with physicians. If the physicians who care for our population are not healthy, how can they provide the best care? We need to set the example for others to follow.

Lessons From the Heart
Question: What organ does the heart feed first?
Answer: Itself

The American Medical Association (AMA) Code of Medical Ethics on the topic of Physician Health and Wellness states, "Physicians have a responsibility to maintain their health and wellness for the safety and effectiveness of the medical care they provide."

> However, physicians are not taught how to maintain their own health and wellness. And this is my "why."

This is why we are here together.

Whatever you're currently facing, I promise it can get better. By reading this book and putting the tools I offer into practice, you will learn to prevent and relieve your stress and completely turn your health and happiness around, just like I did. In fact, I geeked out and did a blood test to find out my telomere length, which can show your age. What was the result? At 52 years old, my telomere length measured 36 years old, so I am actually 16 years younger at the cellular biologic level than my chronologic age! If I can transition from someone so sick, beaten down, and suicidal to a happier, healthier, and more energetic and fulfilled version of myself, so can you!

IMAGINE THIS

What would it feel like to wake up with energy every morning rather than counting down the hours until you can go back to sleep? How would it feel to be calm, relaxed, and efficient throughout your workday and to be present and focused with your family and friends and really *(really)* enjoy your time off? What if people loved being around you again? What if your aches, pains, and other symptoms decreased or were eliminated completely? What if you finally stopped overeating, overdrinking, or "over-anything" that you are using to escape your chronic stress? What if you looked in the mirror and really loved who you saw?

What you're imagining *is* possible.

Feeling stressed is optional!

How to Use This Book

K.I.S.S.

A few years ago, when my home was being constructed, my general contractor got a text from a subcontractor in answer to his question, and all it said was "K.I.S.S."

He asked me if I knew what it meant and I just shrugged. So what did we do at the same time? Googled it! And then we laughed together—K.I.S.S. stands for "Keep it simple, stupid," and reportedly originated in the U.S. Navy. I like to say, "Keep it simple, silly," because it is gentler and I wasn't allowed to call anyone stupid as a kid. So let's stick with silly.

I never forgot that phrase, and I use it as a reminder regularly (and I try to remember to be kind to myself and call myself silly, not stupid)!

Because I know how busy you are.

And I know you feel time-crunched.

And I know how much you want and deserve to feel better.

I designed this book with all of this in mind, to teach you how to feel better quickly and effectively *all by yourself*, to remind myself to keep it simple, silly, and to make it as easy as possible for you in two ways:

- Stress-free snacks—small bites of information
- Providing *what*, *why*, and *how* each stress-relieving tool works

Stress-Free Snacks

I have deconstructed my whole-person approach to prevent and reverse the symptoms of chronic stress into short, actionable bites of information, which I call stress-free snacks, as they apply to the six pillars of Lifestyle Medicine.

What, Why, and How

Most of us know we need to stop stressing so much, eat better, exercise more, get more sleep, improve our social lives, and decrease or stop using risky substances as an escape. But most of us have never been taught what practices we can use to feel better, why we need to do these things, the science behind why they work, and how to do them. This last piece is especially key. Teaching you this hands-on component allows you to experience firsthand what you're learning.

I have found my unique way of teaching to be extremely effective, incorporating this *what*, *why*, and *how*:

1. *What* it is you are learning
2. *Why* the tool works and *why* it is important for your health and well-being
3. *How* to do it through hands-on learning

Throughout this book, you will have the opportunity to practice many effective tools along with me, using several different formats:

through video, audio, and worksheets, which you'll use to build your own personal "stress-relief toolbox." Then you can utilize and implement your tools whenever you need them for whatever situation may arise.

YOUR STRESS-RELIEF TOOLBOX

In every chapter of this book, you'll find tools related to what you're learning so you can immediately relieve your stress. Each tool includes a QR code to a short, actionable video or audio file to help you learn by practicing along with me, so that I can be with you 24/7, whenever you need me.

You'll also find a complete list of QR codes with all of the links I've included at the end of the book (page 219) for easy reference, as well as additional resources (page 217) and citations (page 233) for further information if your brain is craving more (like mine does!).

For each of the tools I present, I'll share why they work and how to practice them. To get the most from this book, I'd encourage you to take off all the hats you wear (if you are a physician, then take off your physician hat) and adopt a beginner mindset. This will keep you curious and open-minded to facilitate your learning and personal growth.

As you read, take each chapter one step at a time, *in order*, rather than skipping around. You can always go back to something you've learned previously, but the chapters are intentionally crafted in a specific order, building on one another to help you get the most effective results.

I'd like you to think of the tools that I'm sharing with you as a buffet. I invite you to "taste" each one and see which ones work best for you. Just like a buffet, some things taste amazing and some things don't taste good at all. That is okay because we're all wired a little differently, and what works really well for one person may not work as well for another. Pick the tools you like—there are no right or wrong answers! You're building *your* personal stress relief toolbox, so only keep the stuff that works for you.

Your Favorites

When you find tools that you really like, put them somewhere you can access them quickly and easily. For example, this can be on a sticky note by your bathroom sink or by your computer monitor, on your night table, or in the notes section of your phone. I'd recommend including your top three go-to tools on this list. I've also created a worksheet to help you remember the tools you've learned.

Toolbox Worksheet

You can use the questions below to help you keep track of your favorite tools. For a downloadable version of this worksheet, go to StressFreeMD.net/worksheets

Name of tool:

How does it make me feel?

Did I find this helpful?

If yes, when can I practice this tool to strengthen it and increase its effectiveness?

In what situations is this tool most helpful?

Where can I access it if I need a reminder? (Where have I written it down or documented it? What is the URL, page #, etc.?)

©Stress Free LLC

MIND OVER MATTER

> "Whether you think you can,
> or you think you can't, you're right."
>
> —Henry Ford

Thought Work Video

Before diving into this book's content, it's important to acknowledge the immense power of your thoughts and the basics of thought work to elevate your success in effectively applying what I will be teaching you in this book.

The thought work I've learned, implemented, and now teach through life coaching is based on evidence-based cognitive behavioral therapy (CBT).

How does it work?

1. You have a thought about a circumstance.
2. That thought drives your feelings and emotions.
3. Your feelings and emotions determine your actions and inactions.
4. Your actions and inactions create the results in your life.
5. Your results ultimately reflect your original thought.

So, in other words, your *thoughts* create your *results*.

When you are feeling stuck, it's essential to do the thought work to get to the root cause of what you're feeling, which is a thought that doesn't serve your greatest good.

HOW TO USE THIS BOOK

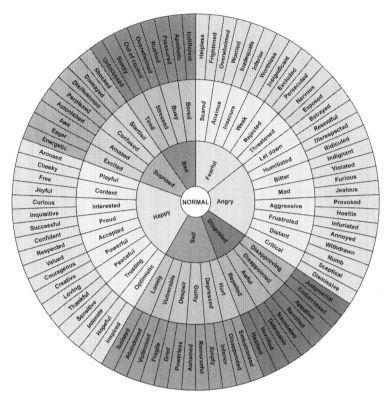

The feelings wheel can be a helpful tool to identify your emotions. Use this diagram whenever you need help clarifying your feelings for any of the exercises in the book.

Thought Work Questions

- What is the exact circumstance or situation?
- What thought am I having about this circumstance or situation?
- What is the main feeling or emotion created by that thought?
- What actions and/or inactions are being driven by that feeling or emotion?
- What is the result from the actions and/or inactions?

Once you identify the underlying thought that doesn't serve you, you can then come up with another thought that serves you better, which will drive the feelings, emotions, and actions needed to get to the result to move you forward.

5 STEPS TO EFFECTIVE BEHAVIOR CHANGE

Behavior Change Video

Now that you understand the power of your thoughts, let's dive into how you can effectively change the behaviors you desire to change.

Have you ever wanted to make a change in your life, say that you are going to do it, maybe even try to do it, and then it just doesn't happen?

I get it. That used to be me. I would have the best intentions—the idea sounded great in my head—but I'd never get lasting results. Or I'd even fail to start because changing my habits was too overwhelming. Does this sound like you?

If so, you are not alone. Did you know that the vast majority of New Year's resolutions fail? An article in *Forbes* says over 80%[3] of people have great intentions, but here is the missing piece: they don't have clear ideas about *how* to achieve their goals. And this isn't just around New Year's. It happens all year long.

So what does effective behavior change look like? It's important to understand that there's more to changing your behavior than just setting a goal. A big part of why people fail at their goals is that they haven't done the *necessary preparation* beforehand to ensure they're ready to take on the changes the goal will require. This is the key—the missing piece. This is the part of creating effective behavior change you were never taught.

What I have come to understand is that there are multiple steps you need to take even *before* writing out your goals and to-do lists. Once I began implementing these steps for myself and my clients, *voila*! My behaviors began to change successfully. And so did the behaviors of my clients.

I have implemented K.I.S.S. here, making it simple by breaking this method down into 5 key steps for you to follow and implement your effective behavior changes.

> I created a 5-step worksheet for you to follow, which you will find at the end of each chapter.
>
> **Step 1:** Identify the behavior to change.
>
> **Step 2:** Determine where you are on the Transtheoretical Model of Change.
>
> **Step 3:** What's your confidence level?
>
> **Step 4:** What's the importance level?
>
> **Step 5:** Set your CALMER goal.

STEP 1

Identify what behavior you would like to change.

STEP 2

Identify where you are on the Transtheoretical Model of Change, which was developed by Dr. James Prochaska.

In the transtheoretical model, there are 5 different levels:

1. **Precontemplation** – You don't believe that you need to change.

2. **Contemplation** – You're thinking about making a change within the next 6 months.
3. **Preparation** – You're aware of the need for change and plan on taking steps within 1 month. During this phase, you may set a goal and write out the steps you need to take.
4. **Action** – You've started making a change but have been doing it for less than 6 months and haven't yet reached your goal.
5. **Maintenance** – You've reached your goal and have sustained the desired behavior for more than 6 months.

These levels apply to any behavior change you want to make, whether that's *stopping* a behavior—such as overeating, drinking, smoking, over-scrolling on social media, yelling and screaming (yes, I have had clients who make this goal)—or *adding* a behavior—such as reading more books for pleasure, working out, getting outside in nature, implementing the stress relief tools in this book—or any other goal that requires you to change your behavior.

In order to make meaningful change, you *first* need to identify *where* you are in these 5 stages. To make an effective behavior change, you need to be at least at the preparation stage. If you're not, ask yourself why. Do the thought work from the previous lesson to identify what's getting in your way and what needs to change in order to reach the next level.

STEP 3

Identify your confidence level in your ability to achieve the goal. Ask yourself this:

"On a scale of 1-10, how confident am I that I can succeed at making this behavior change?"

In order to succeed at making a change, your confidence level needs to be at least a 7 out of 10. If you are feeling lack of confidence, there is a thought that is driving that feeling. That thought is what keeps you from taking action and sets you up for disappointment and failure.

If you're below a 7, ask yourself why and listen to the answer. Do the thought work:

- What thought am I having that is driving my lack of confidence for this behavior change?
- Is that thought true? Is it really true? (Be honest here. Frequently, the thought is not true and is full of self-doubt or negative self-talk.)
- Would other people say it is true? (It can help to see yourself through the eyes of others.)
- What thought do I need to have instead to increase my feeling of confidence to a 7 out of 10 or greater?

Write down the thought you need to have where you can see it and say it over and over again to yourself, until you really believe it and can elevate your confidence level to at least a 7.

STEP 4

Identify the level of importance this behavior change holds for you:

Ask yourself, "On a scale of 1-10, how important is this behavior change to me?"

Like your confidence level, the importance level of the behavior change needs to be at least a 7 out of 10 for success. If you ranked the importance of the change less than a 7, ask yourself why. Do the thought work:

- What thought am I having that is driving my feeling of a lack of importance for this behavior change?
- Is that thought true? Is it really true? (Be honest here. Frequently, the thought is not true and is full of self-doubt or negative self-talk.)
- Would other people say it is true? (It can help to see yourself through the eyes of others.)
- What thought do I need to have instead to increase my feeling of importance to a 7 out of 10 or greater?

Write down the thought you need to have where you can see it and say it over and over again to yourself, until you really believe it and can elevate your importance level to at least a 7.

STEP 5

Once you are in at least the preparation stage and are at least a 7 out of 10 for both confidence and importance, you are ready to create your goal. The word CALMER is an acronym to help you easily remember how to set your effective behavior change goals.

CALMER GOALS

C: Clear – Be as clear and detailed as possible when describing what you want to achieve.

A: Assessable – You can assess if there has been any change in your behavior using concrete measurements.

L: Limited – Your goal has a limited time frame and scope, including a beginning and end date.

M: Meaningful – Your goal is meaningful and applicable to your life, and you understand why you want to achieve it.

E: Exciting – You feel excited to achieve your goal and know you can maintain motivation over an extended period of time.

R: Reachable – Your goal is not too much of an ask and is something you know you can really achieve.

THE 1% BETTER RULE

I know that this may seem like a lot. But like anything, with repetition and consistency, it will become natural and easily integrated into your life. So that it feels less overwhelming, I encourage you to focus on becoming *just 1% better* each day. Start each day by asking yourself, "How can I be just 1% better today than yesterday?" Just 1%. The little changes are truly the big changes.

In each chapter:

- Practice the tools.
- Pause and reflect on how each tool felt for you.

- Fill out your tool worksheet.
- Add the tools that you want to remember to your toolbox (page 35).
- Read, digest, and absorb the content.
- Complete the behavior change worksheet.
- Apply your CALMER goals.
- Determine how you can improve by just 1% today.

1

Pillars of Lifestyle Medicine

"The part can never be well unless the whole is well."

—Plato

> **TOOL: CLEANSING BREATH**
>
> The cleansing breath is usually the first calming breathing tool I teach because it's very accessible, easy to understand, and works quickly. You can share it with your patients and the others you care about in your life. This tool can be used anytime, anywhere.
>
> Consider starting an appointment with you and your patient taking a few cleansing breaths *together* as a way to co-regulate your emotions. If you're stressed out during the workday and are about to go into a patient's room, lead your patient through this cleansing breath as a quick reset. It will help both you and the patient better utilize the short time you have together by calming, grounding, and bringing you both into the present moment, making the visit much more effective, efficient, and meaningful.

Let's try it together now. Use the QR code below to access the video tutorial or follow the steps below.

1. Find a comfortable sitting or lying down position. If you would like, remove your socks and shoes and if sitting, feel your feet touching the ground. Soften or close your eyes if that feels okay for you.

2. Inhale through your nose and lift your shoulders up toward your ears. Feel your shoulders lifting and the contractions in your shoulder muscles.

3. Open your mouth and exhale, lowering your shoulders and feeling them move downward and the de-contractions in your shoulder muscles.

4. Repeat the cleansing breath three to five times or as many times as you'd like.

5. Pause for a moment and notice how you're feeling.

6. Fill out your worksheet for this tool. (StressFreeMD.net/worksheets)

7. If you enjoyed this tool, add it to your toolbox. (Page 35)

Cleansing Breath Video

MY GROSS STORY

Do you want to hear a gross story about my first year of medical school? You probably do. One morning, while in a gross anatomy lab, something *disgusting* happened that would change the trajectory of my life forever. While dissecting a cadaver, I placed my hands inside the abdomen and I felt something sharp on my gloved finger. I quickly pulled my hand out of the cadaver's body and was horrified to see that my glove had been sliced open! (My skin was scratched, but luckily, it hadn't broken the skin.) I looked back into the cadaver's body to identify the cause and found it was a sharp, hard substance along the inner lumen of the abdominal aorta. I called over my anatomy professor for some help and learned that what sliced my glove open was a piece of atherosclerotic plaque in the aorta. Pretty disgusting, right? Big whoa!

That moment made me deeply curious about what caused that plaque deposition in the first place and if there was a way we could prevent it. Of course, my brain then began to wonder whether that plaque was inside me. You may be thinking that now too, right? I get it.

Plaque Be Gone

This is pretty scary: Research has identified arterial plaque formation as early as adolescence from poor dietary patterns (for example, eating donuts and Pop-Tarts for breakfast).

Plaque blocks the flow of your blood in the vessels, which means the cells and organs in your body cannot get the nutrients they need. For example, when this occurs in your heart, it results in a myocardial infarction (MI), also known as a heart attack. When it occurs in your brain, it results in a cerebrovascular accident (CVA), also known as a stroke. So you can imagine that my mind was blown when I dove into the incredible research of Dr. Dean Ornish[4] on reversing heart disease. He was the first pioneer to prove that your body can reverse this damage and remove the plaque in your arteries—yes, actually remove it!

As a Diagnostic Radiologist who loves imaging, I was beyond amazed to see the before and after coronary angiogram images from this research initially showing plaque narrowing coronary arteries and blocking blood flow, followed by a significant decrease in the quantity of plaque with improved blood flow. So amazing!

You may be thinking now, *How do I prevent and eliminate any plaque in my body?* Well, I am glad you asked! This is just one of the many wonderful transformative effects you can create by making 6 key lifestyle behavior changes. Dr. Ornish's Spectrum program for reversing heart disease is based on lifestyle changes and is the only program of its kind utilized for reversing heart disease that Medicare covers. As a board-certified Lifestyle Medicine physician, I am beyond excited to share these lifestyle behavior changes with you!

WHAT EXACTLY IS LIFESTYLE MEDICINE?

Check out these startling stats:

Chronic diseases are incredibly common, accounting for 80% of U.S. healthcare costs, and 80% of chronic diseases are related to lifestyle choices. What does this mean? That 80% of chronic diseases are actually *preventable!*

PILLARS OF LIFESTYLE MEDICINE

> So what is *Lifestyle Medicine*? Lifestyle Medicine is an evidence-based, board-certified medical specialty that uses therapeutic lifestyle interventions as a primary modality to prevent, treat, and sometimes reverse symptoms, illnesses, and diseases. Lifestyle Medicine focuses on 6 key pillars:
>
> 1. Stress management
> 2. Healthful nutrition
> 3. Restorative sleep
> 4. Regular physical activity
> 5. Positive social connections
> 6. Avoidance of risky substances.
>
> Lifestyle Medicine also includes 1 unofficial pillar:
>
> 7. Nature as medicine*
>
> *Nature has been described and reported as the unofficial 7th pillar of Lifestyle Medicine by my amazing friend and colleague Dr. Melissa Sundermann, also known as Doctor Outdoors.

Let me say that traditional Western medicine is truly incredible. Remember I *am* a Western-trained medical doctor and grateful for Western medicine's incredible technology. But Western medicine has become a disease management system, managing, for example, common illnesses such as hypertension, diabetes, and heart disease predominantly with medications. However, Lifestyle Medicine focuses on the opposite end of the medical spectrum by getting to the root cause of an issue.

In Lifestyle Medicine, the patients are considered part of the healthcare team, and they're in the driver's seat with the physician right next to them, actively making decisions together, learning, and coming up with a plan together. Lifestyle Medicine utilizes a team-based multidisciplinary approach to help patients effectively succeed in their goals and treatment.

Patients are acknowledged in how they feel about what's happening and are given information to understand it. They learn the tools they need to take control of their lifestyle and their health, and even if they fall off track with their treatment, they have the knowledge they need to get back on board again.

These changes can frequently decrease or eliminate the need for medications and prevent unnecessary therapies, surgeries, or other procedures. The ability to take your health into your own hands by making key lifestyle changes is incredibly empowering. It puts you in charge of your own health and well-being.

YOUR GENES ARE *NOT* YOUR DESTINY

Let's talk prevention. It's so encouraging to know that the positive lifestyle changes you make today will impact you in the years to come and prevent disease. I frequently hear "Heart disease runs in my family," "Diabetes runs in my family," and "High blood pressure runs in my family." The amazing thing is that *only* 10% of disease is a result of genetics alone, and 90% is based on epigenetics. It is within that 90% where you can make an incredible impact on your health. Just because you have a family history of a particular illness does not mean that you are automatically doomed to suffer from that illness. By taking your health into your own hands and implementing positive lifestyle behaviors, you can keep those genes of concern from expressing themselves, essentially keeping them turned off. Your genes are *not* your destiny!

LIFESPAN VERSUS HEALTHSPAN: HOW DO YOU WANT TO SPEND THE LAST DECADE OF YOUR LIFE?

Lifespan = how long a person lives on this earth

In 2014, for the first time in history, research showed that children's life expectancy, their lifespan, was *shorter* than their parents.[5] What is the primary cause of this increase in mortality? Unhealthy behaviors that lead to chronic disease.

Healthspan = how long a person lives on this earth *in good health*

On average, the last decade of a person's life is not spent in good health—it is spent in poor health, suffering from chronic disease. There is so much talk about wanting to live longer. Your goal should not be to simply increase your lifespan, but to *increase your healthspan* as well—the amount of time you are able to spend a healthy and enjoyable life. This is accomplished by implementing positive lifestyle behaviors. I know I want to be able to keep up with my grandchildren someday! How about you?

The Lifestyle Medicine goal:
Add years to your life and add *life* to your years.

STRESS LESS AND ADD LIFE TO YOUR YEARS

You may be thinking, *I can't add one more thing to my jam-packed life*. I get it. I know what it feels like to think you don't have time to do anything "extra." At times it seems that even using the bathroom or eating are considered luxuries. At least, that was the unwritten message we were given during medical training. How crazy is that?

When clients tell me they don't have time, I reply, *"You are right!"* Why? Because not taking care of yourself robs you of life, both lifespan and healthspan.

That's why the tools I will teach you are designed for the busy lifestyle of a physician. Think of them as small, digestible bites of actionable information, like stress-free snacks!

I invite you to practice the tools in this book whenever you have a short break or *while doing other things* so you don't have to carve a chunk of time out of your day. For example, you can use many of these tools and practices *while* driving, charting at your computer, walking between rooms, scrubbing before a case, watching TV, folding the laundry, walking the dog, emptying the dishwasher—you get it? When you utilize your tools *while* doing other things, you are not carving additional time out of your already super-packed day!

Throughout each chapter in this book, I'll cover a variety of stress relief tools as they relate to each Lifestyle Medicine pillar. The more you practice the tools, the greater your neuroplasticity (new neural pathway formation), and the quicker your tools will work. Think of repetition and consistency as your friends. They are essential to making the tools the most effective they can be for you to feel better all by yourself, whenever you need to use them.

It is time to create a life you don't need a vacation from!

2

Stress Less, Relax Better

> "You are the sky.
> Everything else is the weather."
>
> —Pema Chödrön

TOOL: STRAW BREATH

When you inhale, your sympathetic nervous system increases your heart rate, which is stimulating. When you exhale, your parasympathetic nervous system decreases your heart rate, which is calming. Focus on the exhale component of your breath to feel calmer.

You can naturally lengthen your exhale by breathing out through a smaller hole than you breathe in.

Let's try it together now. Use the QR code to access the video tutorial or follow the steps below.

1. Find a comfortable sitting or lying down position. If you would like, remove your socks and shoes and if sitting, feel your feet touching the ground. Soften or close your eyes if that feels okay for you.

2. Inhale comfortably through your nose.

3. Purse your lips and create a shape with your mouth as if you were drinking out of an imaginary straw. Then slowly exhale through that imaginary straw at the rate that would cause the flame of a candle to flicker on a birthday cake without blowing it out. Allow your exhale to be as long as comfortably possible without force, just invitation of length.

4. Repeat straw breath 3-5 times or as many times as you would like.

5. Pause for a moment and notice how you are feeling.

6. Fill out your worksheet for this tool. (StressFreeMD.net/worksheets)

7. If you enjoyed this tool, add it to your toolbox. (Page 35)

Straw Breath Video

SEEING THE FOREST

Getting to the root cause of my vast number of what seemed like disconnected symptoms took many years. None of the medical specialists I consulted could help me. Know that I don't blame them one bit. It really wasn't their fault. They just hadn't been taught in their training how to diagnose and help me.

I imagine going through medical training to be similar to wearing blinders like a horse or gazing through a microscopic lens, allowing only a narrow viewpoint, unable to see the forest through the trees. In healthcare, it's imperative to remove the blinders and look through the macroscopic lens to see the *whole forest,* because stress affects the *whole person* and can manifest in a wide variety of symptoms. And because stress is such a common problem among healthcare professionals and worldwide, it is beyond crucial that we make its prevention and relief top priority.

After removing my own blinders and gazing through the macroscopic lens, I finally saw the forest. It was only then that I was able to figure out on my own that chronic stress was causing all of my symptoms as well as how to alleviate them. If I hadn't made my own diagnosis and learned how to self-regulate and bring balance back to my whole self, I doubt I would still be here today. I saved my own life. Literally. And I'm so incredibly grateful to be here today to share what I have learned with you.

WHAT IS STRESS, REALLY?

Myth: Stress is a normal and unavoidable part of life. It's part of what physicians signed up for and they shouldn't complain about it but instead put their heads down and just keep going.

Truth: Stress is common but can be prevented and relieved by making key lifestyle choices.

So what is stress anyway? In order to understand stress, let's start by defining it. First off, not all stress is bad. Really! It is usually thought of as negative feelings and emotions, but there is more to stress than that. Stress is broken down into 3 main categories:[6]

1. **Eustress** is positive stress. It's motivating and inspiring, like falling in love, being excited to give a meaningful presentation, accepting an award, or writing this book for you.

2. **Neustress** is neutral stress. It doesn't affect you deeply or personally. It's generally information you perceive as inconsequential or unimportant to your life, such as hearing about an earthquake in another country. You know that's not a good thing, but it doesn't affect you much, and you keep going about your day without pause or distraction.

3. **Distress** is negative stress. It's what most people simply call *stress* (and what we will be referencing when we talk about stress throughout the book). It comes from information we perceive as threatening, which can be real or imaginary. Your brain doesn't know the difference between real and imaginary threats and responds the same way to both.

Furthermore, **distress** is broken down into *acute* and *chronic*.

Acute distress is short term. It comes intensely and disappears quickly. An example might be when someone cuts you off in traffic, but you rapidly adapt and are able to continue to drive.

Chronic distress is long term and can come quickly and intensely, or it can come on slowly, build up, and linger. A common cause of chronic lingering distress comes from job stresses.

Acute stress plays an important role in keeping us adaptable to our circumstances, but with chronic stress, the body is constantly on guard, thinking that there's danger even when there isn't. Chronic stress is the really damaging type of stress because our bodies aren't meant to be in distress all the time. It drains our resources and causes dis-ease, which leads to disease.

So now that you understand the different types of stress, what causes stress in the first place? Stress is caused by a stressor. Stressors alter the balance of the body, the homeostasis. Stressors also come in several different categories, including the following:

1. **Psychological stressors** are thoughts, beliefs, and perceptions. They come from the messages our brains send us, consciously or subconsciously.
2. **Physiological stressors** are things that happen to our bodies, such as illness, infection, disease, and even hunger.
3. **Social stressors** are things that affect our lives, such as personal conflicts, financial insecurity, and significant life changes such as moving or getting married.
4. **Bio-ecological stressors** include weather, pollution, food additives, and other chemicals you may put into your body.

What is the most common type of stressor?
Psychological.

What is the most common type of psychological stressor in adults?
Job stress.

> Stress has been categorized as the world's top health problem, and in the United States, up to 80% of primary care visits are related to stress.[7]

This statistic's most concerning part is that the number of care visits related to stress has increased significantly in the last few years, by at least 10%. More symptoms related to stress are arising, causing more and more patients to seek physician help.

Remember physicians are patients, too.

Look at this list of stress symptoms and see if you see yourself in any of it or maybe *all* of it. I know I have.

STRESS SYMPTOMS

- Palpitations
- Dyspnea
- Sweating
- Irritability
- Tiredness/fatigue
- Loss of appetite/overeating
- Dizziness
- Nausea
- Headaches
- Excessive worry
- Tremors
- Unusual emotional feelings/mood swings
- Difficulty sleeping
- Night sweats
- Indigestion and/or diarrhea
- Irritable bowel syndrome (IBS)
- Feeling unwell or unable to relax
- Low self-esteem
- Depression

If it isn't bad enough that chronic stress makes us feel awful, the health effects of stress are *incredibly* damaging and frightening.

HEALTH EFFECTS OF STRESS[8]

- Impaired immune system
- Increased inflammation
- Decreased bone density
- Problems with memory
- Increased appetite
- Weight gain
- Fat deposition in the abdomen
- Increased insulin resistance
- Increased blood sugar
- Increased cholesterol
- Increased triglycerides
- Increased blood clotting
- Impaired wound healing
- Poor sleep
- Increased sensation of pain
- Increased fatigue
- Worsening of mood
- Adoption of less healthy habits

CUTTING LIFE SHORT

And it doesn't end there! Let's talk about telomeres. Telomeres are the protective ends of your chromosomes. Their length determines your longevity. You can think of them like the protective plastic pieces on the ends of your shoelaces that prevent them from fraying, called aglets (great word to know if you like word games).

Telomerase is the enzyme needed to add the nucleotides, the building blocks, to the ends of your chromosomes to create telomeres. With chronic stress, telomerase is blocked and telomeres prematurely shorten, which speeds up the aging process and causes you to live a shorter life. It actually decreases your longevity. And I know you didn't come this far to only come this far. Yikes!

But guess what? Dr. Dean Ornish's research identified that although stress prematurely shortens telomeres, it's also reversible.[9] You can build them back up!

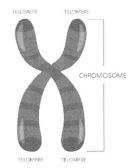

Stress management is critically important. Uncontrolled chronic stress has a domino effect:

- Chronic stress is an etiological (causal) factor in certain medical conditions such as heart disease, stroke, and diabetes.
- Chronic stress precipitates medical conditions in at-risk populations such as obese individuals.
- Chronic stress is a negative prognostic indicator in chronic health conditions like cancer.

So it's vitally important to learn how to prevent and relieve the chronic stress in your own life and the lives of others.

PHYSICIAN STRESS

Work-related stress is the top stressor for most adults in the U.S., and for physicians, the workplace can be extremely stressful. Physicians' jobs tend to be highly demanding, and the prominent mentality that we're taught from the very beginning is to just "suck it up." You're taught to put your feelings aside and keep moving on to the next task, that you have no right to complain.

In the book *The Body Keeps the Score*, Bessel van der Kolk, M.D. reveals how the stress and emotions you push away, ignore, and fail to process sit in your body. And over time, this makes you sick, causing "issues in your tissues."

Stress robs you of joy. We're facing an escalating epidemic of physician burnout, worsened by the COVID pandemic. Medscape 2023 reported that 53% of physicians were burned out in 2022, up from 42% in 2018,[10] with the AMA reporting in 2023 that 63% of physicians were burned out.[11] That's a significant rise, from approximately one in two physicians to two in three physicians. Burnout is defined as being composed of three main components: emotional exhaustion, cynicism, and lack of self-worth. Our own Surgeon General has declared burnout among healthcare workers to be a national crisis. The key etiology is chronic stress.[12]

The lack of self-worth associated with burnout comes from not feeling valued, which can lead to a lack of self-care. When you're chronically stressed, taking care of yourself is even more difficult. You develop poor habits: not eating right, not exercising, sleeping poorly, engaging in little social connection, and even drinking alcohol, self-medicating, or choosing other escapes as a temporary Band-Aid to cover up unwanted feelings and emotions.

Over time emotional and physical exhaustion leads to cynicism, a feeling of not caring, even though you're a caring person. This is the exact opposite of the feeling physicians had when filling out their medical school applications. One of my physician clients during a coaching session said, "Medicine trains us *away* from ourselves." I had to hold back tears when I heard that, as I felt it with *every* cell in my body. Some of the kindest, most caring physician clients cry to me, sharing that they feel absolutely numb, uncaring, and impatient when their patients are describing their symptoms.

Physicians are struggling with their mental health, including depression. According to Medscape's 2023 report, 23% are depressed, and colloquial depression (feeling sad) is on the rise, increasing by 3% over this past year. *Forbes* reported that by 2025, 75% of healthcare workers will leave the profession.[13]

THE PROBLEM BEGINS WITH OUR SEEDLINGS

The problem of chronic stress for physicians begins as early as medical school—at what I call the "seedling level." Research compared two groups of students who just graduated college: those who were going to medical school and those who were not. The study found that those going to medical school had *lower* rates of burnout and depression symptoms and *higher* quality of life (QOL) scores compared to age-similar college graduates not going to medical school.[14] So medical students begin medical school with *better* mental health indicators than age-similar college graduates in the general population. This tells us that the training process and environment contribute to medical students' mental health deterioration.

Other studies show that through the course of medical school, 50% of medical students burn out,[15] up to 30% become depressed, and 10% have suicidal ideation,[16] all while still attending the medical school they were so happy to be a part of in the beginning.

Professionalism is a core competency for physicians. Research comparing 7 U.S. medical schools showed that burnout was associated with self-reported unprofessional conduct and less altruistic professional values, such as caring for the underserved.[17]

Unfortunately, these statistics only worsen during internship. Suicidal ideation doubles from 10% to 20% during the first year of residency. Suicide is the number one cause of death in male residents and the number two cause of death in female residents after cancer.[18]

So why is it that medical students begin medical school healthier and happier than their non-medical school peers, and then quickly become burned out, depressed, and suicidal?

Physicians are taught to put everyone else first. They're taught that necessities like eating and going to the bathroom are luxuries.

Medscape reports that only 40% of physicians care for themselves on a regular basis.[19] When I look back at my medical journey, I can think of several times that this applied to me. During my internship, when I was sick with the flu, I remember my resident hooking me up and running IV fluids into my arm between patient admissions. And I wasn't the only one doing that. It was "normal."

With my first pregnancy, during my fellowship, for several months I had a heplock (capped-off IV) in my arm with an IV pole next to my bed, running IV fluids all night at home and between patients while at work. I was working two to three 36-hour shifts per week with multiple episodes of vaginal bleeding. I would frequently ultrasound myself to make sure all looked okay with my fetus and then I kept on going. I worked when I was pregnant with both of my children up until the time I was in labor and could work no more.

My physician husband was with me overnight while I was in labor during our first child's birth but was called back to work in the morning immediately afterwards. It was even worse following the delivery of our second child, as he was required to work and was not even allowed to drive us home from the hospital. I had to call on a family member for assistance. Again, this was considered normal. Looking back now, I still can't believe it!

THE PROBLEM

So what is the problem? I see it as twofold:

1: The Healthcare System

I am frequently told by my physician colleagues and clients, "The healthcare system is just broken."

My response is *"Yes, you are so right."* That is one of the sources of the problem. The healthcare system *is* sadly broken. And I don't know if it will be fixed during our lifetime. I can't fix it, and probably neither can you.

But here is what we *can* fix: the humans who work within that system.

2: The Human

The second source of the problem is that the people who work within it are not well and have not been taught tools to help themselves.

While I may not be able to do much to fix the healthcare system, what I *can* do is help at the level of the human. My deep passion is to do just that: teach you how to be the happiest, healthiest version of yourself, independent of the healthcare system or anything else going on within or around you. I want you to be able to find calm in the chaos. Even if the healthcare system can't be fixed in my and your lifetimes, your wellness can't—and shouldn't have to—wait until it is.

A Note About Hope

Know this: Hope is *not* an adequate plan. "I hope things get better soon." "I hope I feel better soon." No. It just doesn't work that way. Albert Einstein is often attributed as saying, "No problem can be solved from the same level of consciousness that created it." Whatever you're struggling with, you can't merely hope to get better. If *you* don't change, nothing will.

STRESS AND THE NERVOUS SYSTEM

To understand how stress affects the body and what you can do to improve your stress, it's important to understand what's happening in your nervous system when you experience stress.

In chronic stress, the stress response outweighs the relaxation response in function, like a scale out of balance. What controls this balance or imbalance in your body? Your nervous system.

There are two main components of your nervous system:

1. The **central nervous system**, which includes your brain and spinal cord
2. The **peripheral nervous system**, which is broken down into the **somatic** and **autonomic** nervous systems

The **somatic nervous system** is voluntary. So when you do a bicep curl, you communicate to your arm through the somatic nervous system and tell it to make a fist with your hand, flex your elbow, and curl in your arm.

The **autonomic nervous system** controls the automatic functions of your body, such as your heart beating and your lungs breathing. You are not telling your heart to beat or your lungs to breathe. They just do. I remember thinking that autonomic sounded like *automatic* way back in medical school. That is an easy way to remember the difference between these two components.

The autonomic nervous system is further broken down into **sympathetic** and **parasympathetic** components.

The **sympathetic nervous system** is responsible for the stress response. You often hear the stress response called the fight-or-flight response. It is also known as the fight, flight, freeze, fold, and fawn response as many more components have been identified since its original discovery.

The **parasympathetic nervous system** is responsible for the opposite effect—the relaxation response, a state of deep rest that helps to bring balance, homeostasis, to the physical and emotional responses to stress through the vagus nerve. The vagus nerve (cranial nerve 10) is the main nerve of the parasympathetic nervous system. The word "vagus" means "wanderer," in Latin, and the vagus nerve wanders from your brain through your thorax, pierces your diaphragm, and goes into your abdomen and pelvis. It innervates many key organs along the way.

The stress and relaxation responses are the key opposing functions of your autonomic nervous system. You need these two components to be friends and work together to keep you in homeostasis or balance. Like pedals in a car, you can think of your stress response as representing the gas pedal and your relaxation response representing the brake pedal. You want both pedals to be working with—not against—each other, just like you would in your car.

However, when the stress response is winning and is taking over, your sympathetic nervous system is essentially in overdrive. You can think of it like flooring the gas pedal, "pedal to the metal." That's what it's like when you're chronically stressed.

ALL BODY PARTS ARE NOT EQUAL

What is this? Kind of looks like **one of** my oral board examiners—ha! **Well, it** is our old friend homunculus! Notice how the homunculus depicts large hands, mouth, tongue, and face. The homunculus is a geographic map of the body in the brain. Notice how **each** of your body parts are not equally **mapped** in your brain. Certain body parts take up more "real estate" in your brain, such as your hands, mouth, and tongue, indicating that more neural pathways are involved in these parts of the body.

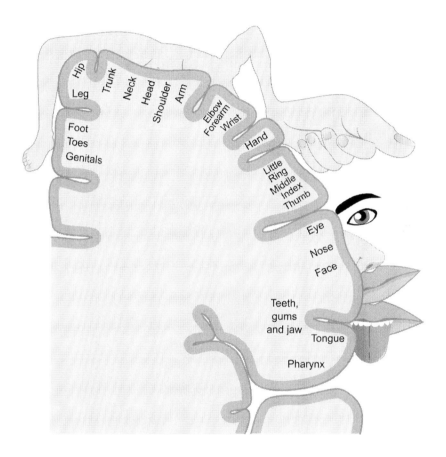

Here you can see the homunculus draped over your motor and somatosensory cortex. Look how much more brain tissue is taken up by your hands, mouth, face, and tongue than the rest of your body.

Understanding the parts of your body that take up more real estate in your brain can be helpful in learning techniques to relieve stress. Working with your hands, mouth, tongue, and face uses more neural pathways and allows you to feel calm more quickly.

HOMUNCULUS EXPERIENTIAL LEARNING

With one finger, gently stroke the back of your forearm. Now do the same thing on your palm. Now your lip. Did you notice the difference? Your palm and lip are so much more sensitive, right? Look how skinny the forearm is in the diagrams on the prior two pages. There are many more neural pathways involved when sensing your lip and palm than your forearm. We can utilize this anatomy and physiology to our advantage by focusing on both the vagus nerve and the larger mapped areas in your brain such as your hands, mouth, and face, to initiate a rapid effective relaxation response to interrupt and regain control of the stress response and allow you to quickly feel calm.

Homunculus Video

2 KEY CALMING TOOL COMPONENTS

To feel calmer quickly, utilize these two components:

1. Focus on the larger mapped areas in your brain: hands, face, mouth, lips.
2. Increase your vagal tone by activating the vagus nerve.

Let's practice incorporating these two key components.

One way to activate the vagus nerve is through creating sound. Have you ever noticed feeling calmer when you sing or hum? I like to add humming to some of my breathing tools because it helps to feel calm faster for two reasons:

1. The vagus nerve partially innervates your larynx (voice box), and you stimulate that nerve when you create sound.
2. The vagus nerve's right and left divisions travel on either side of your neck in the carotid sheaths and are stimulated by sensing the vibrations of sound in your neck.

TOOL: CLEANSING BREATH WITH SOUND

Let's try this together:

1. Follow the steps to practice your cleansing breath. (Page 45)
2. This time when you exhale, add an *ahhh* sound.
3. Repeat 3-5 times or as many times as you would like.
4. Pause for a moment and notice how you are feeling.
5. Fill out your worksheet for this tool. (StressFreeMD.net/worksheets)
6. If you enjoyed this tool, add it to your toolbox. (Page 35)

Cleansing Breath With Sound Video

TOOL: STRAW BREATH WITH HUG

When you focus on utilizing the parts of your body that take up more real estate (space) in your brain, you feel calmer more quickly. These parts include your hands and mouth.

Let's try this together:

1. Follow the steps for Straw Breath. (Page 53)
2. This time, gently cross your arms over your body as if you are giving yourself a well-deserved hug.
3. As you practice this breathing tool, feel your hands touching your body and your body touching your hands. Feel your body moving forward and back beneath your hands and arms with each breath.
4. Repeat this breath 3-5 times or as many times as you like.
5. Pause for a moment and notice how you are feeling.
6. Fill out your worksheet for this tool. (StressFreeMD.net/worksheets)
7. If you enjoyed this tool, add it to your toolbox. (Page 35)

Straw Breath With Hug Video

BOTTOM-UP, TOP-DOWN STRESS RELIEF

How do you feel? I hope calmer! If so, you just experienced what I call "bottom-up" stress relief. Bottom-up means that to feel calmer, you work *first* through your body.

Let me explain.

Your mind is extremely busy. You have around 60,000 thoughts a day (and many of them are not so nice and are on repeat). Often these not-so-nice thoughts lead to stress-related symptoms. I like to think of this as "living between your ears," totally disembodied. When you are mind *full* (two words) it is very difficult to be mindful (one word) and effectively listen, understand, and work with your thoughts.

Here's the amazing thing: you can't think and feel at the same time. Really! You can't think a thought and feel a feeling simultaneously. You are either doing one or the other. So when you put your focus on sensing a feeling in your body, you can come out of your busy, thinking mind and back into your body—become reembodied. Your body relaxes, and you create more space in your mind. Then you can begin focusing on your thoughts with the "top-down" approach, which utilizes life coaching skills.

THE OVERARCHING EFFECTS OF STRESS

Understanding chronic stress is foundational to improving your health and well-being in two key ways:

- Bidirectionality of stress and the Lifestyle Medicine pillars
- Bidirectionality of your body and mind

Bidirectionality of Stress and Lifestyle Medicine Pillars

Stress and the other pillars of Lifestyle Medicine have a bidirectional relationship. What do I mean by that? Stress causes unhealthy food choices, decreased sleep, lack of exercise, lack of social connection, decreased time in nature, and partaking in unhealthy habits such as using risky substances and other escapes. And when you are eating poorly, exhausted, not moving your body, isolated, and utilizing risky substances, that all leads to feeling stressed.

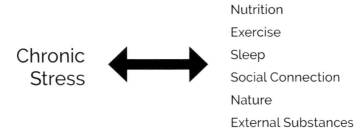

Here's more on the specific ways the 6 pillars have a bidirectional effect on your stress:

1. **Nutrition** – When you're stressed, your body craves immediate energy because it thinks you are in an emergency situation. It causes you to crave unhealthy foods that are high in saturated fats and added sugar, which then causes even more stress and anxiety for two reasons: one, you are upset with yourself for eating such junky food, and two, this junky food has been shown to increase stress, anxiety, and depression. Eating unhealthy foods makes you feel worse. Food creates mood.

2. **Sleep** – When you're stressed or anxious, you don't sleep well, which may include difficulty both falling asleep and staying asleep. And when you don't sleep well, it causes exhaustion and more anxiety and stress.

3. **Exercise** – When you are stressed, you are less likely to move your body and exercise regularly. Exercise is a wonderful stress reliever. Without exercise, you don't have an outlet for your stress, you may gain weight, and your negative thoughts about yourself for not exercising cause even more stress.

4. **Relationships** – When you're stressed, you're not showing up as your best self in your relationships. You may remain isolated from others, fail to socially connect at all, or you may be reactive, saying or doing things you wish you could take back. Lack of social connection causes feelings of isolation and loneliness, increasing stress.

5. **Risky substances** – When you're stressed or anxious, you may turn to self-medicating with risky substances to numb these unwanted feelings, such as alcohol or recreational drugs. Dependency on external substances causes a poor self-image and increases your stress.

6. **Nature** – When you are stressed, you are less likely to spend time outside, which leads to greater stress and anxiety. Hippocrates said, "If you are in a bad mood, go for a walk. If you are still in a bad mood, go for another walk." Why? Because research shows that being in nature and breathing in phytoncides (scents given off by plants) decreases the stress hormone cortisol, heart rate, blood pressure, and anxiety.

Bidirectionality of the Body and Mind

In addition to the bidirectionality of stress and the Lifestyle Medicine pillars, there is also bidirectionality between the body and mind. A thought can cause a feeling in your body. Your body can also sense a feeling first and then send a signal to your brain. This happens when you get a "gut feeling." Millions of neurons make up your gastroenteric nervous system, also known as your "second brain." You know when you get an uneasy feeling about a situation in your gut, right? You walk into a room and something just doesn't feel right and you have a "gut feeling." Then your brain follows with a thought recognizing that something isn't right.

This also happens with your heart. HeartMath studies have shown that your heart actually sends more signals to your brain than your brain sends to your heart.[20] Your heart (like your gut) can sense a feeling about a situation before you have a thought about it. Amazing!

The Stress Umbrella

Although all the pillars of Lifestyle Medicine interact and directly affect one another, I see stress as the umbrella under which all other pillars live. Since stress is America's number one health problem and causes 80% of symptoms, it really is the overarching pillar encompassing all of the others.

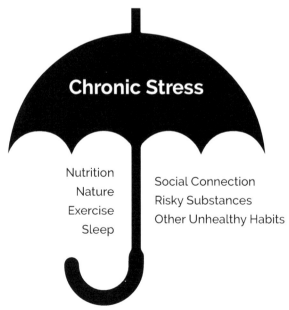

Before I began to heal from my chronic stress, I was already eating a healthy diet and exercising a lot. However, it wasn't until I started relieving my stress that all the symptoms I was experiencing started improving and eventually disappeared. None of it got better with pills, physical therapy, occupational therapy, acupuncture, massage, chiropractic care, mental health care, or anything else I was doing to treat it because I wasn't getting to the *root cause* of my issues, which was chronic stress. Those modalities were wonderfully palliative, giving me temporary relief, but they were not curative.

Once I learned tools to bring my nervous system into homeostasis, I felt calmer, began to sleep better, and woke up with energy. I noticed that I was more connected with people, including my kids. I was more connected with myself and understood what was really important to me. I stopped drinking alcohol and consuming caffeine. I felt well enough that I didn't need any of the pills I'd been taking.

I learned that when my stress was relieved, the other Lifestyle Medicine pillars fell into place. It would have been impossible to do all of those other things if I didn't fix the stress first.

I've seen the same thing happen over and over again with my clients.

BODIES RESPOND TO STRESS DIFFERENTLY

All bodies and minds are different, and we can't predict how they'll react to stress. For me, it was several symptoms in my body combined with negative thought loops that all resolved completely as I learned how to relieve my stress. I've had many clients with symptoms they couldn't get rid of who finally felt better after working with me, when they learned how to relieve their stress using my bottom-up, top-down approach.

It is so interesting where stress "lives" in your body. One of my favorite yoga therapy mentors (also an orthopedic nurse) used to say that her mother-in-law lives in her left big toe, because whenever she was with her mother-in-law, her left big toe would be excruciatingly painful.

As for me, I get a weird, chronic tugging pain in one spot in my left lower back. I tried everything imaginable for years and could not get rid of it. On the first morning of iRest® meditation training, I was feeling this tugging in my left lower back while sitting and listening to the opening lectures. Following the lectures, we were guided through a meditation, and I was wowed when I got up off the floor and the tugging in my back was totally gone! I put on my curious lens, had an aha moment, and recognized that this is a place where stress lives in my body! Now, whenever I feel that tugging, I don't pop Advil or Tylenol or seek any help from outside therapy. I just know it's my body reacting to a stressor, and with my stress-relieving tools, I can relieve it all by myself. No medical treatment needed!

Learning the signs of stress in your own body can be invaluable. When that tugging pain returns for me, I know there's nothing wrong with me—it's just my body saying, "Knock-knock. Time for you to chill out a bit and take care of yourself."

Knowing what is happening with your body and nervous system puts you in the driver's seat. It's like the check engine light—maybe your gas cap is a little loose, and all you need to do is simply tighten it.

TIME TO TRANSFORM!

For a downloadable version of this worksheet, go to StressFreeMD.net/worksheets

BEHAVIOR CHANGE: STRESS

What stress-related behavior would you like to change?

Identify your current stage in changing the behavior you identified above and circle your answer:

1. Precontemplation – *You don't believe that you need to change.*

2. Contemplation – *You're thinking about making a change within the next 6 months.*

3. Preparation – *You're aware of the need for change and plan on taking steps within 1 month. During this phase, you may set a goal and write out the steps you need to take.*

4. Action – *You've started making a change but have been doing it for less than 6 months and haven't yet reached your goal.*

5. Maintenance – *You've reached your goal and sustained the desired behavior for over 6 months.*

If you are not at least at stage 3, do the thought work necessary to get there. (Pages 38-42)

On a scale of 1-10, how confident are you that you can make the desired change? Circle your answer.

          1 2 3 4 5 6 7 8 9 10

On a scale of 1-10, how important is it to you to make the change? Circle your answer.

          1 2 3 4 5 6 7 8 9 10

If you scored lower than a 7 for either confidence or importance, do the thought work needed to score higher.

If you scored a 7 or above, you're ready to set your CALMER goals.

CALMER GOALS

C: Clear – Be as clear and detailed as possible when describing what you want to achieve.

A: Assessable – You can assess if there has been any change in your behavior using concrete measurements.

L: Limited – Your goal has a limited time frame and scope, including a beginning and end date.

M: Meaningful – The goal is meaningful and applicable to your life, and you understand why you want to achieve it.

E: Exciting – You feel excited to achieve your goal and know you can maintain motivation over an extended period of time.

R: Reachable – Your goal is not too much of an ask and is something you know you can really achieve.

What can you do to improve your stress by 1% today?

3

Stress Less, Eat Better

"Let food be thy medicine and medicine be thy food."

—Hippocrates

> **TOOL: EMPTY WRAPPER SYNDROME**
>
> Have you ever reached into a bag of chips or tried to take a bite of an energy bar only to find that there was nothing left? This used to be me. I call this "empty wrapper syndrome," mindless eating when your brain is someplace else—mind *full* (two words), not mindful (one word), and focused on anything and everything except your food. For example, this can happen when you are eating while working at your desk, walking in between patients, watching TV, or driving your car, and you are completely dissociated and unaware of what you are doing. Sound familiar?
>
> Mindless eating leads you to eat too quickly and overeat, which then causes poor digestion, abdominal distention and pain, and weight gain. What happens next? For many people,

this leads to frequent negative self-talk, which only exacerbates the whole situation and ultimately causes you to feel stressed.

I invite you to try this mindful eating tool, which you can do *while* you are doing activities that might cause mindless eating. It takes no added time out of your day and can give you a much better overall eating experience.

1. Choose a small, solid piece of food that you enjoy.
2. Find a comfortable seated position.
3. If you have to open a package or unwrap the food, notice the sound.
4. Place the food in the palm of your hand.
5. Look at the food. Notice its shape, color, and size.
6. Feel the contact the food makes with your hand.
7. Pick up the food with your fingers, feel it being held by your fingers, and bring it toward your nose. Notice how it smells.
8. Place the food between your lips and sense the texture.
9. Place the food onto your tongue (don't bite it), roll it around, feel the texture, and taste it.
10. Take a single small bite and again, roll it around, feel the texture, and taste it.
11. Repeat this again and again until the food is completely chewed, paying attention to noticing the texture and taste.
12. Then slowly swallow and sense the food moving to the back of your mouth and throat.

13. Now has that food tasted better than ever before?
14. Pause for a moment and notice how you are feeling.
15. Fill out your worksheet for this tool. (StressFreeMD.net/worksheets)
16. If you enjoyed this tool, add it to your toolbox. (Page 35)

Mindful Eating Video

WHEN NUTRITION IS SAD

Do you remember the gross story I told you in the first chapter about dissecting a cadaver my first year in medical school, during anatomy class when the plaque from my cadaver's aorta cut my glove wide open?

Well, in the back of my mind, I always knew that diet played some kind of role in health, but I didn't truly understand the dramatically damaging effects it could have until that aha moment. This piqued my curiosity (my doctor-to-be brain wanted to learn so much more), so I began to deepen my knowledge of the etiologies (causes) of atherosclerotic plaque and how to prevent and even reverse it.

It was that single anatomy class experience that drove me to pivot and begin my transition away from eating animal products. This was for three main reasons: my own health, the health of the animals (this one is the easiest to comprehend), and the negative effects animal farming has on our planet, including carbon dioxide (CO_2) emissions which harm the atmosphere; wiping out land in order to feed livestock; and ultimately, the climate change epidemic. Despite my vegan diet, however, I still had a lot of digestive problems. I was frequently constipated and dealt with a significant amount of abdominal pain and distention after eating.

It wasn't until I dove into studying the nutrition pillar in Lifestyle Medicine that I found I had much, much more learning to do. I was surprised to learn that just because I wasn't eating animal products didn't mean I was eating healthy. What was I doing wrong? I was still eating highly processed, nutrient-poor foods full of chemicals, sodium, saturated fats, and added sugars. For example, I didn't know that processed vegan turkey with vegan cheese in a sandwich wasn't really healthy. I was eating veggie dogs and veggie burgers and all sorts of processed stuff. I thought I was doing so well, but I came to realize that I was only exchanging one type of unhealthy food for another, having made a lateral move when it came to my own health.

Looking back several decades, I can't remember a single nutrition lecture during medical school. I asked my med school classmates to make sure it just wasn't my memory lapsing, and they all confirmed that we had no nutrition education. And when I asked my much younger physician clients the same question, I received the same answer. Physicians are just not educated about nutrition. Learning about glucose in the Krebs Cycle absolutely does not count. I didn't know that foods with 25-letter ingredients were bad for me. I just thought, "It's not an animal, so it's probably okay." I was blown away by how much more there was to learn.

What defines an unhealthy diet? According to the World Health Organization, an unhealthy diet is one that is based on processed foods with added fat, sugar, and salt, along with animal products rich in saturated fats. An unhealthy diet is low in vegetables, fruits, legumes, whole grains, nuts, and other high-fiber foods. This is describing the standard American diet (SAD), which most Americans are consuming. And yes, this is *really sad!*

The SAD diet breaks down to 63% processed foods, including added fats, sugar, and refined grains; 25% animal products, such as meat, dairy, and eggs; and 12% plant foods, such as vegetables, fruits, legumes, whole grains, nuts, and seeds. So only 12% of the SAD diet is composed of healthy plants.

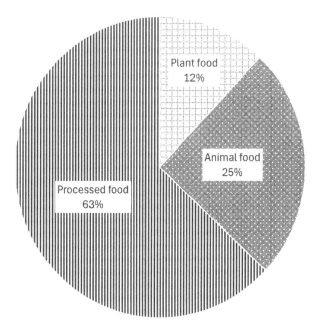

Graphic produced using data from USDA, Economic Research Service, 2009. https://www.ers.usda.gov/publications/EIB33; https://www.ers.usda.gov/publications/EIB33; retrieved from "Brain Food: How does nutrition affect the developing brain, in turn affecting the experience of stress" https://cam1084.wordpress.com/2014/03/26/the-sad-standard-american-diet/

The SAD diet is the leading cause of chronic illnesses, diseases, and disabilities including weight gain and obesity issues.[21] According to the Cleveland Clinic,[22] 74% of Americans are concerned about their weight. Are physicians concerned about their own weight? As it turns out, yes. Research shows that 50% of physicians are trying to lose weight and 31% are trying to maintain weight, so more than 80% of physicians are concerned about their weight, which is an even *higher* statistic than the general public.[23]

The good news is that simple dietary changes can make a big difference in your health outcomes. In fact, substituting just 5% of dairy in the standard American diet with plant-based foods results in a 24% decrease in cardiovascular disease.[24] That doesn't mean you should stop there—you'll continue to see more benefits, the more plants and fewer processed foods you eat.

You know what's really exciting? The changes that occur when you switch to a healthy diet happen remarkably quickly.

WHAT IS A HEALTHY DIET, ANYWAY?

Lifestyle Medicine focuses on healthful nutrition and encourages eating as many plants as possible in their *whole* state. This is known as a whole food plant-based approach to nutrition, often shortened to WFPB, a pattern of eating that includes fruits, vegetables, grains, beans, legumes, nuts, and seeds that are nutrient-dense and minimally processed, and it is the opposite of the standard American diet. The WFPB diet contains *no* animal products and also doesn't include any highly processed foods.

I came to understand the difference between the unhealthy vegan diet I'd previously utilized, full of highly processed foods, and a WFPB healthful diet. Vegan doesn't necessarily mean healthy at all. You can be vegan while still consuming an unhealthy diet.

You might be wondering what is a highly processed food? Here is an example using an apple: If you have an apple, that's a whole food. Once you make it into applesauce, it's less whole. And apple juice is even less whole than applesauce. You can process it even further to make a fruit roll-up or a gummy bear. The whole apple, however, is the best, most healthful way to eat it. The more you process it, taking elements away, the less nutritious it gets. By the time it becomes a piece of candy, potentially dangerous chemicals have been added and most, if not all, the nutritional benefits of the apple have been lost.

So when deciding on what is healthy food and what isn't, I come back to this K.I.S.S. quote:

> "Nothing bad added, nothing good taken away."
> —Michael Gregor, M.D., FACLM

HOLD UP!

Now let me pause here and say that I don't want to scare you away! I don't want you to stop reading! I am not trying to make you give up all of the foods that contain animal products that you love and tell you that you must go full-on vegan. My goal is just to share with you what I've learned and help you add more plants to your plate.

Think of using this terminology to describe the eating pattern you want to achieve:

- Plant-slant
- Plant-forward
- Plant-powered
- Plant-centered
- Plant-strong

> "Eat food, mostly plants, not too much."
>
> —Michael Pollan

HOW I TRANSITIONED

Throughout my nutrition journey, I have learned how to make many easy food switches. I identified the foods I liked and found ways to create or buy healthier versions of them. For example, I stopped drinking processed energy drinks and learned to make my own healthy drinks and smoothies from real, whole foods. I even make my own delicious plant-based milks. So fun!

My focus changed from thinking about sources of single nutrients to the whole food package. I began to ask myself where I could get a better source for all the nutrients I needed.

I began paying attention to food labels and reading the ingredients, becoming aware of added sugars, saturated fats, and sodium content as well as added chemicals. I decided that if I couldn't pronounce or spell an ingredient then I probably shouldn't be eating it!

I noticed that eating healthier led to many physical benefits including improved digestion, normal bowel movements, nourishing sleep, and better skin and hair quality, to name a few.

As I changed my diet, I also began to feel stronger and have more energy on a daily basis. Even at the gym, I felt more like Wonder Woman (no, I wasn't wearing the outfit!) than Rip Van Winkle with the amount of strength I had gained.

Eating healthier also led to improvement in my emotional health. I became less agitated and anxious, less reactive, and calmer and more patient. I also felt my previously depressed mood elevate.

Of course, there were days when I wasn't perfect. It's normal to have days when you want to eat junky stuff. But on those days, I noticed that I felt sluggish and didn't have the energy and focus I usually had. I wasn't as creative or motivated, and my mood wasn't as good. It's incredible how much better I feel when I eat healthier.

Think of your body like a car that needs specific gas to function properly. If you put regular gas in a car that needs high octane, it doesn't perform well, putters along, and drives unsteadily—this once happened to my car, which required high octane gas, when I was on a road trip in a rural area, visiting colleges with my son, and only regular gas was available. That's just like what your body does when it doesn't get the proper nutrients that it needs.

THE FOOD-MOOD DYNAMIC

> ### YOU ARE WHAT YOU EAT
>
> Have you ever heard the old Cherokee story about the two wolves?
>
> An old Cherokee was teaching his grandchild about life. "A fight is going on inside me," he said to his grandchild. "It is a terrible fight and it is between two wolves. One is evil, full of anger, envy, sorrow, regret, greed, arrogance, self-pity, guilt, resentment, inferiority, lies, false pride, superiority, and ego. The other is good, full of joy, peace, love, hope, serenity, humility, kindness, benevolence, empathy, generosity, truth, compassion, and faith. The same fight is going on inside you, and inside every other person, too."
>
> The grandchild thought about it for a minute and then asked his grandfather, "Which wolf will win?"
>
> The old Cherokee simply replied, "The one you feed."

FOOD AFFECTS MOOD

You might think your mood is generally caused by a situation you are experiencing or a thought you are having—angry about this, happy about that. But did you know that the food you eat actually directly affects your emotions and how you are feeling? I found it absolutely fascinating to learn how strongly food and mood are connected, each affecting the other.

According to *Lancet Psychiatry*, "Although the determinants of mental health are complex, the emerging and compelling evidence for nutrition as a crucial factor in the high prevalence and incidence of mental disorders suggests that *diet is as important to psychiatry as it is to cardiology, endocrinology and gastroenterology*."[25]

So the old saying "you are what you eat" is true! Eating the wrong foods can be quite damaging to your emotional and mental well-being. Research shows that consumption of fast foods, processed foods, fried foods, meat, dairy, fatty foods, refined sugar, and trans fats is associated with increased rates of depression and anxiety.[26]

Fiber, which is *only* found in plant foods and not animal foods, is crucial to your emotional and mental health and well-being. Why? Because fiber feeds not only your body but your gut microbiome, allowing for a healthy gut (eubiosis), and 90% of your serotonin and 50% of your dopamine, your good feeling hormones, are formed in your gut.

Due to the standard American diet, 95% of Americans are below *the recommended daily allowance for fiber.*[27]

An unhealthy gut microbiome (dysbiosis) is associated with many illnesses and diseases, including mental illness such as anxiety, depression, bipolar disorder, schizophrenia, Alzheimer's, and autism.[28]

On the flip side, a plant-based diet high in whole, unprocessed fruits and vegetables is associated with a low incidence of depression and anxiety.[29]

In addition, omnivores (people who eat animal and plant foods) who were placed on a vegetarian diet (no meat, fish, or eggs) showed improvement in mood scores with significant improvement in depressive symptoms *in just two weeks*![30]

People who eat more plants have higher *eudaimonia*, the feeling of meaning and purpose in their lives. A healthy plant-based diet improves creativity, productivity, and focus and is associated with lower stress levels. Overall, it creates a greater sense of vitality and improved quality of life.[31]

MOOD AFFECTS FOOD

When you feel stressed out, what foods do crave? Do you find yourself reaching for lettuce, carrots, and celery? No! It's probably more like ice cream, chips, candy, French fries, and chocolate, right? As we discussed back in chapter 2, when you feel stressed, your body seeks out immediate energy in the form of sugar and fats, so you are more likely to reach for unhealthy foods high in sugar and fats. But eating those foods will actually worsen your mood, not help it.

FOOD INQUIRY

I invite you to take a moment to think about how you have felt after eating certain foods:

- How do you feel after eating different types of foods?
- Do certain foods make you feel sluggish, tired, anxious, or depressed?
- Do you experience abdominal bloating and pain when you eat certain foods?
- Do certain foods make you feel constipated?
- Do certain foods lead to good bowel movements?
- Do certain foods make you feel calm, happy, and energized?

What did you learn about yourself?

Moving forward, continue to be mindful and pay particular attention to how certain foods make you feel. You may even want to keep a journal if that helps to keep track of what you learn.

FOOD AS YOUR FRIEND

Dr. Koushik R. Reddy is the first interventional cardiologist to become certified in Lifestyle Medicine, and I absolutely love his scrub top, which says it all. It has the medical caduceus symbol in the middle with a carrot to the left and a cardiac stent to the right. Underneath, it reads, "I have a carrot and a stent—you pick!"

As I mentioned earlier, you really are what you eat. Your body can't perform all of its vital functions if it isn't given the necessary ingredients.

Eating a healthy diet can result in a great number of benefits to your health.

Determines Your Epigenetics

Earlier in this book, I mentioned that your genes are not your destiny and that only 10% of your risk of disease is genetic, while the other 90% is epigenetic, related to your lifestyle behavior choices. Nutrition plays a vital role in your epigenetics.

Epigenetics are the ways in which the expressions of your genes change as a result of your lifestyle behavior choices. You're born with certain genes but you can change the way they're expressed. For example, you may have a gene that leads to cancer, but that doesn't mean you'll necessarily end up getting cancer,[32] because that gene may not be expressed or turned "on." When you are living a healthy lifestyle, certain genes will stay turned "off" and not express themselves. But unhealthy lifestyle choices such as poor nutrition can turn "on" those damaging genes, leading to illness. Eating a healthy diet improves your epigenetics to keep those unwanted gene expressions turned "off."

Prevents and Reverses Chronic Disease

A whole food plant-based eating pattern lowers your overall risk of chronic disease and is even able to help treat and reverse certain types of chronic diseases, such as diabetes type 2 and Alzheimer's dementia.[33]

Lowers Risk of Cancer

A whole food plant-based eating pattern lowers the risk of cancer because in addition to the epigenetics component described above, it minimizes gene mutation. An unhealthy diet causes inflammation in your body and genetic mutations, where genetic expression is altered and genes are no longer expressing the way they should, allowing for cancers to form and grow.

Lowers Total Caloric Intake

When you're eating healthy, you have a lower total caloric intake because you are eating nutrient-dense—not calorie-dense—foods, and your body perceives earlier satiety (feeling full). Eating fiber-rich, plant-based foods expands your stomach much more quickly than eating animal-based or processed foods. When you have fewer feelings of hunger and a smaller caloric intake, it's easier to maintain a healthy weight.

A healthy plant-based diet also improves the efficiency of leptin, the hormone that tells you when you're full, as well as adiponectin, which regulates insulin sensitivity, glucose levels, and lipid metabolism.

Improved HbA1c and Insulin Sensitivity

The level of HbA1c in the blood is used to diagnose diabetes or prediabetes. It evaluates your levels of glucose averaged over the last three months and indicates how well your insulin is functioning. Eating a healthy diet improves insulin sensitivity, keeping glucose levels and HbA1c normal.

Strengthens Immune System

A whole food plant-based diet is rich in antioxidants that reduce damaging free radicals in your body, which lead to chronic illness and disease. Nutrient-rich foods also promote the production of white blood cells that ward off infection.

Lowers Endothelial Injury and Improves Arterial Flow

A healthy diet reduces inflammation in the body. Inflammation causes endothelial injuries—injuries to the lining of your blood vessels—which develop small tears, allowing for plaque deposition. That plaque then builds up and narrows your arteries, and it can eventually block the flow of blood in your arteries, like a piece of fruit can block the flow of your smoothie in your straw. Without adequate blood flow, tissues and organs cannot receive nutrients for function and survival.

Improves Cardiovascular Disease

Cardiovascular disease can also be prevented and reversed through dietary changes, as shown by the research of Dr. Dean Ornish.[34] The country of Uganda has a cardiovascular disease rate of only 9.85% (2017) compared to the global rate of 31.8%.[35] This is largely a result of the fact that the people of Uganda mainly eat a plant-based diet with little to no animal products. Compare that to the standard American diet, which causes extensive cardiovascular disease and many deaths.

Optimizes the Gut Microbiome

Did you know you have 38 trillion organisms living in your gut, but you only have 30 trillion cells in your body? You actually have more bacteria living in your gut than you have human cells in your body! Those bacteria, your gut microbiome, form a protective layer in your gut, which plays an important role in healthy digestion, keeping your immune system strong, producing vitamins such as vitamin K, and regulating your blood sugar.

Your gut also regulates your mood as 90% of the serotonin and 50% of the dopamine—your good feeling hormones—are made in your gut. It's important to protect your gut microbiome by feeding it fiber, because that's what the good gut bacteria eat. Fiber can be found in vegetables, fruits, grains, legumes, nuts, and seeds. *There isn't any fiber in animal products.* Adding more fiber to my diet was an important step in my nutritional transformation.

Decreases Blood Pressure

Many processed foods have a high level of sodium. Sodium causes fluid retention, which increases blood volume and blood pressure.

Lowers Fat and Cholesterol

Animal products are high in saturated fats and contain no fiber. Eating a plant-based diet low in saturated fats and high in fiber decreases your cholesterol level. Research shows that by changing your diet, in just two weeks you can lower your cholesterol in amounts equivalent to the effects of taking statin drugs.[36]

IT'S A FAMILY AFFAIR

I want to share a story with you that blew my mind. One of my clients was a physician mom who came to me for stress and anxiety management. She was like many physician moms I knew—super busy working and taking care of the kids, trying to cut corners and doing things as simply as possible.

When I work with a client I work with the whole person. She described many of the challenges she was facing: She was exhausted, weak, depressed, and overweight. She had a lot of joint pain and gastrointestinal issues. She fed her family a lot of meat (mostly processed) and fast food, which cost her a significant amount of money. Her kids were having some academic issues in school and were acting out at home, leading to frequent fighting. She was screaming at her kids, her husband, and her staff members, feeling out of sorts all the time.

I asked, "Are you okay with talking about your nutrition? I'd love to know what you're eating." And she agreed. I learned that she had been brought up to believe you need to eat meat for protein and dairy for calcium. I knew where she was coming from—those used to be my exact thoughts. I explained to her that diet is the leading cause of chronic disease in the world. Meats are high in saturated fats and processed meats like bacon, hot dogs, and salami are actually class 1 carcinogens, meaning they directly cause cancer. Unprocessed meats are class 2A carcinogens, meaning they likely cause cancer.

There's a big meat industry here in the U.S., so even though the FDA and other major government organizations know that meats can cause cancer and other chronic diseases, it's still very common for people to believe they need to eat meat.

I began to educate my client about how to easily add more plants to her plate and decrease the meat and processed foods. We talked about the kinds of foods her family likes and discussed healthy food swaps and recipes.

She started to make small transitions in her diet and her family's diet little by little. I always encourage taking small steps to keep things manageable.

She tried one recipe at a time and began developing a routine. She stopped ordering out, did more cooking and meal prepping, and noticed that her symptoms were dramatically improving. She felt less tired and more energized. Her joint pain was totally gone. She had stopped going to the gym because her joints hurt so much, but she was able to return to the gym again. Her GI issues—abdominal pain, bloating, diarrhea, and constipation—all went away. She started losing the weight she wanted to lose. Overall, she felt calmer.

After she'd seen so many benefits from changing her diet, she told me something I didn't expect to hear: her kids had started to do better in school. The whole family was getting along better, and they were enjoying more activities together on the weekends.

Previously, her husband and kids hadn't been involved in preparing meals at all. I encouraged her to make it a family thing, and they began spending time on the weekends meal prepping together. It ended up being a really fun family activity. They'd chop vegetables, prepare their overnight oats, and pack freezer bags full of ingredients for slow-cooker recipes to use during the week.

Getting the kids involved allowed her to teach them how to eat healthy but also provided a way for her to connect with them more. She and her husband stopped fighting, and the family was saving money since they weren't eating out.

She was so excited by the changes she'd experienced that she asked her kids' teachers if she could come to the school to talk about nutrition and bring some healthy foods. She set up a time in her local gym to start teaching free classes on nutrition.

It was one of the most incredible transformations I've seen in one of my clients, and speaks to the power of healthful nutrition to positively affect many facets of your life!

> **Myth**: Eating a whole food plant-based diet is too expensive.
>
> **Truth**: A WFPB diet can actually be less expensive than many other diets. It costs a lot more to buy fast food, order out frequently, or buy meat on a regular basis, which actually can cost you your life.

THE LIFESTYLE MEDICINE APPROACH TO NUTRITION

So far you have learned about the importance of eating several types of healthful foods. You may be wondering, "Is possible for me to get enough nutrients from just plants?"

> **Myth**: Eating only plants can't possibly provide all of the nutrients you need, especially protein.

Truth: You can get all of the nutrients you need fairly easily from plants, and there are plenty of plant-based sources of protein.

> "Someone asked me, how could you get as strong as an ox without eating any meat? And my answer was, have you ever seen an ox eating meat?"
>
> *—Patrik Baboumian, vegan bodybuilder,*
> The Game Changers

As a diagnostic radiologist, I am a very visual person and I learn best by seeing, which is why I found it incredibly helpful to have a visual image of how best to set up my plate. I visualize each food category as pieces of a pie. Eating plants in the right proportions is vital to ensure you are getting the right balance of nutrients. In general it is recommended that your plate contains the following:

- ½ vegetables and fruits
- ¼ plant-based protein
- ¼ whole grains

THE WHOLE FOODS PLANT-BASED PLATE

Unlike the plate of the standard American diet (SAD), which has over 60% processed foods and very few plants, the WFPB plate, per the American College of Lifestyle Medicine, is composed entirely of plant-based foods and contains very little, if any, processed foods.

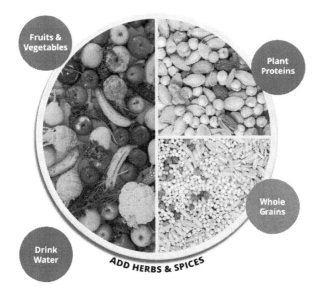

Your fruits and vegetables can be eaten raw or cooked, as long as they are cooked safely. Focus on "eating the rainbow" by including as many different colors of plants as possible. Unlike animal products, plant foods contain more than 100,000 phytonutrients, the natural chemicals responsible for producing different colors in plants, which have antioxidant and anti-inflammatory properties that protect against major chronic diseases.

Healthy grains should be whole grains, such as quinoa, buckwheat, rice, and even breads and pastas as long as they're made from unprocessed, unbleached flours and don't contain processed ingredients.

Wonderful sources of proteins include legumes, beans, nuts, seeds, tofu, and tempeh.

In addition to the categories of healthful foods on your plate, remember to stay hydrated! Water is another extremely important element of a healthy diet. Humans are predominantly made of water! Learning how to make water taste good with healthy changes made a big difference in my hydration. Not a fan of plain water? I know it can get boring so I love to infuse my water with cut fruit mixed with herbs such as mint and basil. Naturally flavored sparkling water with no added salt is another one of my favorite choices and is a great healthful option.

As physicians tend to be perfectionists (I get it), know that just because the plate image is divided up like a pie chart doesn't mean you have to only color within the lines and make three separate dishes—this image simply describes the proportions of different food categories needed for a healthy meal, and you can get as creative as you'd like with your cooking. The food categories may be combined to meet your proportions. You have permission to have some fun here!

NOT ALL COOKING IS SAFE COOKING

Beyond eating healthful foods in the right proportions, it's important to understand that not all cooking is safe cooking. Healthy foods can become unhealthy foods when cooked improperly.

Oil

What's the first thing you do when you take out a pan to sauté? Pour in some oil to prevent the food from sticking to the pan. I used to do this as well. But oils are calorie dense and nutrient poor, high in fat, and have been shown to cause cardiovascular disease.[37] Did you know that 1 tablespoon of olive oil has 124 calories and 14 grams of fat?! So instead of pouring some oil into your pan, you can simply swap that out with low-sodium vegetable broth or water. This decreases those unnecessary empty calories and fat as well as your risk for illness.

What about when oil is in a recipe for baking? You can swap out oil with apple sauce, mashed avocado, bananas, or pumpkin!

Cooking Methods

Cooking foods at high heat and for long periods of time creates advanced glycogen end products (AGES), which are associated with chronic disease and cancer. They are commonly caused by broiling, frying, and barbecuing. Instead, it is much healthier to boil and stew foods and slow cook at lower heat. This also preserves food nutrients.

WHAT ABOUT SUPPLEMENTS?

Let me share a story. I had suffered from constipation for years. I felt uncomfortable most of the time from abdominal distention and persistent, bleeding hemorrhoids. I was taking a lot of supplements including B12, vitamin D, and calcium to help me get the nutrients I thought I might be missing because of my vegan diet. Following routine labs for an annual check-up, my internist called me, concerned, because my B12 level was through the roof! She had me eliminate all supplements to find a new baseline. You know what happened next? The constipation actually stopped and I began having great bowel movements! Yippee! Why was I always so constipated? Because I was over-supplementing with calcium which can be very constipating. I did it to myself! I'm so grateful for my astute internist.

I'm sharing this story because sometimes we do need supplements. It's important to consult your physician, review your dietary pattern, and have your bloodwork evaluated to determine what's right for your body instead of just piling supplements on for no reason like I did, which can cause more harm than good. Do you have a drawer or cabinet full of "just because" supplements? It may be time to evaluate what you really need and at what dose.

What does an ideal healthful diet look like?

- Whole food plant-based nutrition
- Healthful foods proportioned properly
- No processed foods
- No chemical additives (including pesticides)
- Healthy cooking methods, such as boiling, stewing, and slow cooking
- No high-heat cooking, such as broiling, barbecuing, and frying
- No added sugar
- No trans fats
- Low to no saturated fats
- Supplementing only if needed and at the correct dosage
- Proper hydration

"IT'S TOO HARD"

Okay, I know I've covered a lot of information, and you may be thinking that this is too hard, especially if this is all new to you as nutrition education in medical school and training is usually little to none. (I had none!) But I promise that making the necessary changes is not as difficult as it might seem!

Beware of the physician all-or-none mentality. Remember that focusing on a plant-forward or plant-slanted diet is perfectly okay. You'll get significant benefits by simply putting more plants on your plate and decreasing less healthful foods.

Myth: It's too difficult to maintain a WFPB diet.

Truth: Keeping a WFPB diet is not any more difficult than any other diet. You just need to be organized. (And as physicians, we thrive on structure and organization!)

ORGANIZATION TIPS

Organization helps you deconstruct what appears to be an overwhelming task, and your methodical mind thrives in organization.

- Plan your meals and snacks for the week ahead of time.
- Create your grocery list including quantities of food needed.
- Don't go to the grocery store without a list.
- Buy only what is on the list, and be careful about getting led astray.
- Commit to using all of the items purchased.
- Consider cooking greater quantities and freeze extras in portion-sized containers.
- Prep food ahead of time for the week.
- Make lunches the night before while cleaning up dinner.
- Invite family members to help—make it a fun family activity!

Remember: you don't have to change everything at once. Focus on improving by just 1% each day!

If you're ready to take your diet a step further and want more information, the American College of Lifestyle Medicine has a free *Food as Medicine* online course. It's self-paced and includes a lot of excellent recipes. I have personally tried many of the recipes, and even my family loves them and requests them!

EASY HEALTHFUL RECIPE: ENERGY BITES

Delicious and easy cinnamon energy bites that taste just like an oatmeal cookie! These no-bake bites make the perfect on-the-go snack or afternoon treat. You can even break them up over a green smoothie at breakfast.

Makes 12 bites.

Ingredients

- 6 large Medjool dates, pitted (about ½ cup packed, pitted dates)
- 1 cup rolled oats (uncooked)
- 1 ½ tsp cinnamon
- ¼ cup peanut butter
- 1/8 tsp salt

Instructions

1. If dates are dry, place pitted dates in a small bowl and cover with hot water for 10 minutes to soften. Drain dates well just before using. If they are juicy and soft, skip this step.
2. Add the oats, cinnamon, dates, and salt to a blender or food processor. Pulse until evenly combined but still chunky.
3. Transfer mixture to a bowl and add peanut butter. Stir until well mixed.
4. Use a small cookie scoop or use your hands to roll the dough into balls.
5. Store in an airtight glass container in the fridge.

(Recipe from Food as Medicine: Jumpstart *by the American College of Lifestyle Medicine, https://lifestylemedicine.org/project/food-as-medicine-jumpstart/)*

TIME TO TRANSFORM!

For a downloadable version of this worksheet, go to StressFreeMD.net/worksheets

BEHAVIOR CHANGE: NUTRITION

What behavior related to nutrition would you like to change?

Identify your current stage in changing the behavior you identified above:

1. Precontemplation – *You don't believe that you need to change.*

2. Contemplation – *You're thinking about making a change within the next 6 months.*

3. Preparation – *You're aware of the need for change and plan on taking steps within 1 month. During this phase, you may set a goal and write out the steps you need to take.*

4. Action – *You've started making a change but have been doing it for less than 6 months and haven't yet reached your goal.*

5. Maintenance – *You've reached your goal and have sustained the desired behavior for more than 6 months.*

If you are not at least at stage 3, do the thought work necessary to get there. (Pages 38-42)

On a scale of 1-10, how confident are you that you can make the desired change?

        1 2 3 4 5 6 7 8 9 10

On a scale of 1-10, how important is it to you to make the change?

        1 2 3 4 5 6 7 8 9 10

If you scored lower than a 7 for either confidence or importance, do the thought work needed to score higher. (Page 38-42)

If you scored a 7 or above, you're ready to set some goals.

CALMER GOALS

C: Clear – Be as clear and detailed as possible when describing what you want to achieve.

A: Assessable – You can assess if there has been any change in your behavior using concrete measurements.

L: Limited – Your goal has a limited time frame and scope, including a beginning and end date.

M: Meaningful – The goal is meaningful and applicable to your life and you understand why you want to achieve it.

E: Exciting – You feel excited to achieve your goal and know you can maintain motivation over an extended period of time.

R: Reachable – Your goal is not too much of an ask, something you know you can really achieve.

What can you do to improve your stress with respect to nutrition by just 1% today?

4
Stress Less, Sleep Better

"Beds are wireless chargers for humans."

—Sophie Vertrees (insightful 9-year-old daughter of my friend Amy Vertrees, M.D.)

> **TOOL: 4-7-8 BREATH**
>
> Unlike the tools in other chapters, this tool is designed to make you sleepy. Please try it at night and not *before* reading this chapter, or you won't make it through the chapter before . . . zzzzzz
>
> Let's try it together *when you are ready to fall asleep.*
> 1. Find a comfortable lying-down position. Soften or close your eyes, if that feels okay for you.
> 2. Inhale through your nose for the count of 4.
> 3. Retain your breath and pause for the count of 7.
> 4. Exhale through your nose for the count of 8.
> 5. If this count pattern doesn't work for you, that is okay. You can decrease or increase the numbers to fit your needs, keeping a similar pattern.

6. Repeat this as many times as you would like until you fall asleep.

7. If you enjoyed this tool, fill out your worksheet (StressFreeMD.net/worksheets) and add it to your toolbox. (Page 35) (Do it the next day since you're using it for sleep.)

4-7-8 Breath Video

I'LL SLEEP WHEN I'M DEAD

Many people, especially busy physicians, see sleep as a luxury because that is essentially what we have been taught. They tend to think they can catch up on it on weekends or vacations and believe that is when they *should* be sleeping. I used to see sleep this way, but it is absolutely false. In fact, sleep deprivation is cumulative.

As a long-time Bon Jovi fan, for years I've sung the song lyrics, "Gonna live while I'm alive / I'll sleep when I'm dead." But eventually, I came to understand that without nourishing sleep, I wasn't really living at all.

> **Myth**: Sleep is a luxury, and you can catch up on weekends or vacation.
>
> **Truth**: Sleep deprivation is cumulative and can have devastating effects on your body and mind.

It used to be normal for me to feel exhausted and like a zombie all the time. I would wake up each morning yawning and before getting out of bed, with one eye barely open, count how many hours I had to get through before I could go back to sleep. Do you do this too? I'd ask myself *how* I was going to get through the day, driving an hour and a half to work, working all day, then driving the hour and a half home, putting on my "mommy hat" to take care of my children, cook, help with homework, give baths, read books, then do whatever else needed to be done in the house, and try to chat with my busy physician husband somewhere in there as well.

I somehow managed to hold it together all day at work, dictating all the cases, doing all the procedures, and praying that I wasn't making any mistakes or hurting anyone. I'd get into my car to drive home and explode into tears on my commute from how exhausted I was. I'd shake it off before walking in the house to not upset my family. Then I'd get up to do it again the next day.

My lack of sleep caused me significant anxiety and stress, which then robbed me of even more sleep. I'd lay in bed worrying about going to sleep. Then I'd wake up during the night worried, have trouble getting back to sleep, and wake up anxious about not getting enough sleep. It was a vicious cycle, and it's a common complaint that brings many of my physician clients to me for help.

COME DANCE WITH ME

My sleep transformation began when I started incorporating several stress-management techniques and lifestyle changes into my daily routine. As I began to regulate my nervous system and feel calmer, I could fall asleep with greater ease and decrease the number of times I was waking up in the middle of the night. After a little while, I began to wake up less tired and more refreshed. And it only got better from there.

In addition to utilizing stress-relief tools, I found that I no longer needed to start my day with caffeine, the drug I'd required to keep me going. I didn't even realize I was addicted until one of my yoga therapy mentors, during an evaluation in response to my sleep issues as well as my daytime jitteriness, asked me why I was drinking caffeinated tea every morning. "Are you drinking this because you need the caffeine, or is it soothing to you?"

I didn't know the answer to that right then and there, but I *was* learning about how caffeine is not only a stimulant but causes the secretion of catecholamines, stress hormones, from your adrenal glands, and delays the onset of sleep.

She suggested I swap the morning caffeinated tea for hot water with lemon instead. Once I did the swap, I was able to fall asleep more easily, and I lost the jitteriness and felt so much calmer. It made me realize that I was very sensitive to caffeine, and it was just the warmth of the drink that was soothing to me in the morning—I didn't need caffeine!

Improving my sleep started from the bottom up with the stress-management techniques I was learning. Now that I teach these techniques to my clients, I've seen many transform their sleep by implementing the practices.

One of the most encouraging success stories I've heard was from a military veteran in his 70s. He'd fought in the Vietnam War and was in one of my Veterans at Ease classes, which incorporate yoga therapy and meditation. After class one day, he came to me with tears in his eyes and told me, "I'm finally sleeping, and I haven't slept in about 50 years." I held back my tears. This man struggled with PTSD and cardiac issues and had undergone many surgeries, but by incorporating the stress relief tools I'd taught him at home, his stress significantly decreased, enabling him to sleep.

When you're exhausted and feeling sick due to chronic stress, getting better can seem like an impossible task. But feeling stressed—and sleeping poorly—is optional. The problem isn't that it's hard—the problem is that nobody has taught you how to effectively relieve your stress and improve your sleep.

Myth: I don't have time to sleep.

Truth: Lack of sleep causes decreased focus and productivity. It makes your daily life harder. When you get enough sleep, you can increase your focus and efficiency, which frees up more time for you during your day.

My relationship with sleep has significantly improved as I've become more deeply educated on the topic. I now understand that sleep is an imperative part of self-care. It's a requirement for our health and well-being and ultimately for our happiness. Sleep is truly an amazing friend!

I now love waking up with a smile on my face, feeling energized and ready for the day. I no longer count the hours until I get to go back to sleep. I enjoy starting my day feeling focused, present, and clear-minded. I happily take on the morning with a saying from my friend and mentor Pat Croce, quoting Hafiz: "Come dance with me." This saying reflects what my day will bring and what I will bring to my day. Try it on for size and see how it feels!

THE PHYSIOLOGICAL EFFECTS OF SLEEP (WHOA! SO MUCH GOOD IS HAPPENING HERE!)

When you are asleep, your body is actually not! Incredible physiological changes are taking place.

PHYSIOLOGICAL CHANGES WHEN *DO* SLEEP

Imagine a team of worker bees doing their magic in these ways:

- **Repair and restore DNA**: Mutations occur within your DNA throughout the day. Sleep is responsible for a lot of restoration in your body. Your DNA—your genetic material—is repaired and restored during sleep.
- **Appetite regulation (leptin and ghrelin)**: Sleep is the time for your body to synthesize leptin and ghrelin to regulate your appetite. Leptin is the satiety hormone, which tells you when you are no longer hungry. Ghrelin is the hormone that signals that you are hungry. Good sleep promotes higher leptin levels during the day, which will prevent you from overeating.
- **Growth hormone**: During sleep, you produce growth hormone, which is essential for the health and growth of cells in order for your body to perform all its amazing functions.
- **Insulin regulation**: Sleep regulates insulin, which in turn regulates your glucose level and turns it into energy and nourishment. When you get enough sleep, your blood sugar is more stable throughout the day.
- **ATP synthesis**: ATP is the energy your cells use to function. Its formation is enhanced when you sleep, and it increases your physical energy during the day.

- **Memory encoding**: Your memories are encoded during sleep, so all the things that happened throughout your day and everything you've learned get encoded in your brain while you sleep, so you can remember them later.
- **Lower cortisol**: Your cortisol level is regulated when you get a good night's sleep. Cortisol levels should be highest when you wake up in the morning and throughout the day, they should drop so they're lowest when you fall asleep at night.
- **Lower blood pressure**: Your blood pressure drops when you sleep, which allows the blood vessels to dilate so blood can flow to all of your cells and organs to give them the nourishment they need and to remove waste. This is a vital part of keeping your body healthy.
- **Faster cardiovascular recovery time and improved heart rate variability (HRV)**: Your cardiovascular recovery time and HRV measure how adaptable your heart is. An adaptable heart is a healthy heart and supports a resilient autonomic nervous system that can respond effectively to whatever stressors arise.
- **Apoptosis**: Sleep enhances apoptosis, natural cell death. Natural cell death allows new cells to form. We want cells to die at a certain point because if they don't, they get old and mutate, which leads to cancer.
- **Anti-cancer cytokines**: Anti-cancer cytokines are proteins that float around in your blood and help eliminate cancer cells that shouldn't be there. They're part of your immune system, which is generally stronger when you get a good night's sleep. Sleep is when the body regulates cytokines and TNF (tumor necrosis factor), which helps fight off infections and diseases.

These functions during sleep are vital to your health. When you don't get a good night's sleep, your body cannot perform these functions properly. And sleep deprivation is cumulative, so the more often you don't get enough sleep, the more likely you are to have negative effects as a result.

PHYSIOLOGICAL CHANGES WHEN YOU *DON'T* SLEEP

The negative physiological effects of poor sleep are the opposite of the benefits you gain from good sleep, and they can lead to illness and disease:

- **Decreased restorative processes**: DNA mutations are not repaired.
- **Lower daytime leptin**: Lower leptin can lead to overeating and weight gain.
- **Decreased growth hormone**: Lower growth hormone decreases the health and growth of all cells.
- **Insulin resistance**: Higher glucose levels lead to insulin resistance and lower energy levels.
- **Decreased ATP synthesis**: ATP synthesis is necessary to encode memories, so poor sleep leads to poorer memory.
- **Higher cortisol**: Elevated stress hormones are damaging to the body, causing many symptoms and illnesses.
- **Increased AGE (advanced glycation end product) deposition into the vascular system**: Increased AGE causes oxidative stress and inflammation, which lead to chronic disease.
- **Dyslipidemia**: Dyslipidemia means your fats are not well regulated. You have higher cholesterol levels and the walls lining the vasculature become damaged, where artery-blocking plaque tends to form.

- **Endothelial dysfunction**: This dysfunction causes buildup of atherosclerotic plaque and increasing cardiovascular disease.
- **Increase in obesity**: Obesity is associated with many illnesses and diseases.
- **Metabolic syndrome**: The components of metabolic syndrome are increased abdominal girth, hypertension, elevated cholesterol, elevated glucose, and increased risk of cardiovascular disease, diabetes, and stroke.
- **DM2** (type 2 diabetes)
- **Higher cardiovascular risk and mortality**
- **Increased risk of myocardial infarction**
- **Vasospastic disorders**
- **Reduced BDNF (brain-derived neurotropic factor)**: BDNF plays an important role in learning and memory.
- **Decreased repair and regeneration of nerve tissue**
- **Increased risk of certain disorders:**
  - Depression
  - Bipolar disorder
  - SAD (seasonal affective disorder)
  - PMS (premenstrual syndrome)
- **Worsens symptoms of PTSD (post-traumatic stress disorder) and TBI (traumatic brain injury)**
- **Melatonin suppression**
- **Immune suppression**
- **Increased cancer-stimulating cytokines**
- **Dysfunctional gene transcription and cell cycle**
- **Aberrant DNA methylation**: DNA is not coded correctly as a result of poor sleep.

- **Increased risks of certain cancer types:**
  - Breast cancer
  - Endometrial cancer
  - Prostate cancer
  - Colorectal cancer
  - Acute myeloid leukemia

SYMPTOMS OF POOR SLEEP

While it may take a while for more serious health problems to develop, there are symptoms of poor sleep that can be identified after just a night or two of poor sleep:

- Decreased stamina and increased fatigue
- Difficulty awakening
- Decreased focus and concentration
- Mistakes, errors, accidents
- Decreased presenteeism (loss of productivity in the workplace)
- Increased time to complete tasks, if able to complete at all
- Increased anxiety and fear
- Memory impairment
- Increased appetite and seeking poorer quality and greater quantity of food
- Poor mood
- Reactivity
- Decreased motor skills
- Less social interaction and connection

ADDITIONAL DANGERS OF SLEEP DEPRIVATION

Poor sleep is physically and mentally dangerous. It leads to accidents that affect not only yourself but the lives of others. Research shows that more surgical errors occur after overnight call.[38] According to the National Highway Traffic Safety Administration, the number of car accidents from drowsy driving is similar to the number of car accidents from driving under the influence of alcohol or drugs.[39] Have you ever fallen asleep post-call at a red light? (Full disclosure: I have.)

Another eye-opening fact is that being awake for 24 hours impairs your function equivalent to a blood alcohol level (BAL) of 0.10, which is higher than a BAL of 0.08, which qualifies as legally drunk.[40] When I think about how many 36-hour call shifts we have all done, making decisions with our brains functioning worse than someone who is legally drunk, it's scary.

So, when you understand what sleep does *for* you and what the lack of sleep does *to* you, it's easy to see why it's so important to prioritize quality sleep for your health and for the safety of those around you.

As a healthcare professional, I was blown away when I learned about all the important functions sleep performs. I knew, of course, that it was good for you. I don't remember having any lectures on sleep in my medical training, and culturally, many of us view sleep as a luxury. It's the easiest thing to cut when your schedule is full. I didn't know how damaging the lack of sleep could be! Shout out to all of my sleep specialist colleagues—I now have a newfound utmost respect for you!

> ## HOW ARE YOU SLEEPING?
>
> Let's take a minute to assess the quality of your sleep.
>
> How many hours do you sleep on weekdays?
>
> How many hours do you sleep on weekends?
>
> What is your perceived quality of sleep?

Red Flags That Indicate Poor Sleep

Do you have any of these?

- Sleeping less than 7 hours a night
- Sleeping more than 9 hours a night
- An hour or more difference in sleep duration between the weekdays and weekend
- Irregular sleep patterns
- Irregular sleep duration
- Poor perceived quality of sleep despite enough hours in bed
- Daytime fatigue
- Daytime sleepiness
- Difficulty awakening
- Sleeping more than 8 hours before ideal wake-up time
- Sleep onset is less than 20 minutes after lights out
- Waking less than 7 hours after bedtime
- Poor sleep beliefs, such as "I don't have time for sleep" or "I don't need to sleep"

Did you see yourself in any of these red-flag health scenarios? More than one? If so, no worries! We are going to cover some key things you can do to turn all of this around. The good news is that you can improve your sleep by making lifestyle changes, and in doing so, you'll reduce your stress, which makes it easier to sleep better. Many of my clients have told me that they're now sleeping for the first time in years. And the most surprising thing is that it frequently happens within the first week of us working together.

HOW TO IMPROVE YOUR SLEEP

In addition to utilizing your stress-relief tools, there are several other factors to consider to improve your sleep.

I invite you to put on your science researcher hat, get into the lab, and ask yourself some questions:

1. Do I know why I am not sleeping well?

Can you identify any problems that may be causing you not to sleep well? Let's see if you can get to the root cause of this issue, and then we can find the solution.

2. How many hours am I sleeping?

When looking for problems in your sleeping patterns, start with the amount of sleep you're getting. I don't mean how many hours you spend in bed—the question is how many hours you are actually *sleeping*. Many people get in bed and then do things on their phones for hours. (If you are doing this, you are not alone.)

Getting good sleep is mainly about getting *enough* sleep. The right number of hours to sleep varies from person to person, but on average for adults, it falls between 7 and 9. For some people, 7 is too few, and for others, 9 is too much.

A lot of research has been done on the right amount of sleep for people in different age brackets, but there's controversy over whether those numbers are right for everyone. What it ultimately comes down to is how you feel.

Everyone has what I like to call a "Goldilocks" number of hours of sleep—the amount that feels right to them. That's the number of hours when you wake up feeling refreshed, not tired or groggy. When you get the right amount of sleep, the next day you should feel clear-minded, present, efficient, and responsive (not reactive).

What is your Goldilocks number? Mine is 7 when I am at a well-rested baseline. It's up to you to figure out what your magic number is. Once you know, you should aim for that amount of sleep every night. If you're sleeping less than that, you're not getting enough. And if you're sleeping more, it means your sleep quality is poor and you're too tired. You shouldn't need to sleep more than your Goldilocks number.

3. Is my sleep interrupted?

If you lack sleep due to waking up during the night, ask yourself if you know why.

- Did you wake up because you had to use the bathroom? If so, you may need to stop drinking fluids a few hours before bed.
- Did you wake up because you were worried about something? If so, then addressing that stress before bedtime will be helpful.
- If you're waking up because your body is tense, is it because of your stress or did you do a really hard workout earlier?
- Is there too much light in your room?

- Are you too cold or too hot?
- Is your dog barking?
- Is there anything else you can think of that could be interfering with your sleep?

Here are some additional factors that influence your sleep:

- Daylight
- Blue light
- Temperature
- Exercise
- Food intake
- Hydration
- Caffeine and alcohol
- Bed use

Why are these important? Here are some details.

Daylight

The circadian rhythm is the natural process in your body that makes you want to sleep when it's dark and be awake when it's light. Just like a nocturnal animal is built to be awake during the night, you're built to be awake during the day.

The physiology behind the circadian rhythm is really cool. Part of your retina is for seeing things, and another part of your retina is dedicated just to collecting daylight. When light enters your pupil, it stimulates the retinal ganglion cells (RGCs), which send signals to the suprachiasmatic nucleus (SCN)—known as the central clock of the hypothalamus. The SCN then sends signals to both your pineal gland, which makes melatonin for sleep, and your adrenal gland, which releases the stimulating hormone cortisol.

Through this process, light suppresses melatonin and increases cortisol release, which promotes wakefulness.

It can be tough for people who work the graveyard shift to sleep during the day because of all the light they're exposed to. It messes up their circadian rhythm, and they don't get as much nourishing sleep as they need. That's why it's best to sleep in the dark—your body is wired to sleep that way.

Of course, not everyone can control their schedule to optimize their sleep. But you can take steps to improve sleep by working with your circadian rhythm. Limit light as much as possible at night (or whenever you need to sleep). And when you wake up, get bright light exposure early in the day, especially natural light if possible.

Blue Light

While daylight particularly affects melatonin and cortisol production, other types of light also play a role.

It's best to avoid any kind of screen 1 hour before sleep because screens emit blue light, which your body registers similarly to daylight. Blue light increases heart rate, blood pressure, and core body temperature while suppressing melatonin, which you need in order to sleep.

Chances are you use your cell phone as your alarm. So after you set your alarm, put your phone down on your night table—don't check your email or scroll through social media. Those things are stimulating and can make it hard to fall asleep as the mind becomes busy.

Temperature

Temperature is an important factor in your sleep. To sleep, the body core needs to be cool. Keeping your extremities warm allows cutaneous vasodilation, increasing blood flow to the skin in your arms and legs, which helps dissipate heat from your core.

In order to cool your core and warm your extremities, it is essential to keep your room at a comfortable temperature and keep your body warm with blankets and clothing. Wear socks if your feet tend to be cold. Having a bath or shower before bed can also be helpful—not only does it warm up your body, but the relaxing effects can also help you sleep.

Exercise

Exercise heats your body and is energizing, promoting wakefulness. In order to fall asleep, your core body temperature needs to be cool, so if you exercise late in the day, it can make it more difficult to fall asleep because your body's core is too warm and active to rest.

For this reason, it's best to exercise early in the day to promote wakefulness. In addition, exercise is stimulating and can help you feel more alert and focused even if you wake up a little groggy or have a midday energy dip.

Food Intake

Carbohydrates

Digesting food, particularly digesting carbohydrates, is stimulating. It elevates your glucose levels and heats your core body temperature, which promotes wakefulness. Essentially, it causes your body to kick into gear and get to work, which isn't helpful when trying to sleep.

For this reason, it's great to have a full breakfast with plenty of carbohydrates shortly after you wake up because it will help give you energy quickly. But you should avoid eating heavy carbs late in the day. It's best to have an early dinner and not snack afterward. That includes not sitting in front of the TV and eating snacks after dinner. (I used to do this. What about you?) This will allow your body to have time to digest and cool the core temperature so you can sleep.

Sodium

Limit high-sodium foods, especially in the evening, because they cause vasoconstriction and prevent vasodilation, an important restorative function to dissipate body heat during sleep.

Hydration

Stay hydrated throughout the day to enable vasodilation, increase REM sleep, decrease leg cramps, and decrease thirst in the middle of the night. An added benefit of staying hydrated during the day and not drinking too far into the evening is decreasing the need to go to the bathroom at night, which causes you to wake up, disrupting your sleep.

Caffeine and Alcohol

Caffeine and alcohol are also important factors in the quality of your sleep. Even if you feel like it doesn't affect you, avoid having caffeine in the afternoon or at night. Similarly, avoid drinking alcohol within 3 hours of going to bed, as it's also known to interfere with sleep.

Bed Use

Use your bed for sleep and intimacy only. When you do other things in your bed, your mind begins to associate that space with other activities and thoughts, making it more difficult to relax in bed. You don't realize how many things you do in your bed until you stop doing all those things. It's important to train your brain that your bed is just for sleep, because if you do something like work in bed, then whenever you're in bed, you may still be thinking about work. You want to train yourself that your bed is your happy place so it's easy to relax and calm your mind.

After these factors have been addressed, it's time to improve your transition to sleep.

TOOL: GUIDED MEDITATION FOR SLEEP

1. Find a comfortable lying down position.
2. Ensure you are warm enough (clothing, blankets, room temperature).
3. Relax or close your eyes if that feels okay for you.
4. Listen to this guided meditation with or without headphones. (I love keeping a pair of headphones in my night table drawer for a more quiet, intimate experience.)
5. Fill out your worksheet for this tool. (StressFreeMD.net/worksheets)
6. If you enjoyed this tool, add it to your toolbox. (Page 35)

Guided Meditation for Sleep Video

WHAT DOES GOOD SLEEP LOOK AND FEEL LIKE?

Let's examine what getting good, restful sleep looks like.

Good sleep feels *amazing*! And I can't wait for you to feel that!

- Not tired when you wake up
- Full of energy all day
- Focused and present
- Creative juices flowing
- Productive
- Present

SLEEP TRANSITION ROUTINE: CREATE YOUR DIMMER SWITCH

It'd be nice if we just had a switch we could flip on or off to be awake or asleep, but since we don't, it's important to have a transition routine. A transition routine, or "dimmer switch," helps you practice your healthy sleep habits and wind down for the night so you're ready for sleep. There's also power in routines—your body likes routines and adjusts to them, and practicing the same steps before bed every night can make it easier for your body to remember it's time to sleep. Implement your dimmer switch routine 1 to 2 hours before bed to help you ease into sleep.

Set Your Sleep-Wake Schedule

The first step in establishing your sleep transition routine is setting your sleep-wake schedule so you know when to begin your transition. Your body and mind work best when you know how many hours of sleep you actually need to feel refreshed and ready for the day. Take that number of hours and subtract it from the time you need to wake up in the morning and that becomes the time you need to be asleep in your bed—not the time you get into bed but the time you are *actually* asleep. Then your sleep-wake schedule is set.

Yes, there will be deviations with call schedules, events, weekends, etc., but your body and mind function best when you generally stick to your schedule. Don't worry about being perfect; this is just a guide and it helps your circadian rhythm, your internal clock, to function properly.

Turn On Your Dimmer Switch

One to two hours before bed, begin to implement your sleep transition routine. I have divided the steps into two parts: out of bed and in bed.

Out of Bed

Consider relaxing, non-stimulating activities:

- Take a gentle, slow walk outside, opening up all 5 senses. I love to hear the frogs, crickets, and birds, smell the flowers, watch the ducks, and see the sky change colors as the sun sets as I walk along the mountain paths near my home.

- Do somatic-based gentle yoga to relax muscular tension. Somatic-based is my go-to, and I do it on the floor next to my bed.

- Place your legs up the wall or on a chair to relieve the heaviness of your legs if you were standing for a while. This will decrease your heart rate and blood pressure by stimulating the baroreceptors in your neck (as long as this is medically allowed).

- Try grounding with a calming qigong sequence, a form of exercise and meditation that originated in ancient China. It is sometimes called Chinese yoga and has similar elements to yoga and Tai Chi.

- Turn the lights down in your house and only keep on the minimal light needed. As you turn down the lights, your pineal gland gets the signal through less light being absorbed by your retina that it is nighttime, which means sleep time, and will invite melatonin secretion needed for sleep.

- Put on some comfy clothes. Ditch anything uncomfortable. Take off those work clothes: pantyhose, heels, ties, and belts—yuck! I used to walk around for hours and realize too late that I was still in my uncomfortable "dress-up clothes," as my daughter would call them.

- Take off your socks and shoes and go barefoot. Sense your feet touching the ground, inside or outside. This helps you come out of your busy thinking mind because you can't think a thought and feel a feeling simultaneously.

- Cuddling with another human or pet increases oxytocin, a good feeling hormone.

- Put on soft music, nothing too stimulating. Make sure it is calming. I am very sensitive to sound, and certain types of music agitate me while others relax me.

- Burn a candle or incense. Choose a calming scent that you love. I love vanilla, lavender, and eucalyptus for the evenings.

- Do self-massage with lotion or oil. Use long motions on long bones and circular motions on joints. Add in your feet if you enjoy that as well. I love rolling old (softened) tennis balls on the plantar or bottoms of my feet.

- Take a warm bath or shower to aid in cooling off your core by driving the heat out through your extremities through vasodilation.

In Bed

- Stay warm. Use blankets, clothing, and socks.
- Read in bed, but choose something not work-related or stimulating. Read a real book, nothing with blue light that will suppress your pineal gland's melatonin production.
- Place your legs up on the backboard of your bed (as long as this is medically allowed).
- Practice calming breathing tools such as cleansing breath, straw breath, or 4-7-8 breath.
- Focus on your gratitude and wins. Place a small notebook and pen by your bed and take a moment to write down 3 things for which you are grateful and/or 3 wins. Remember that nothing is too small. Your mind's default pathway naturally gravitates to what is going wrong instead of what is going right. When you take time to focus on what you are grateful for and the wins in your life, your good-feeling hormones, serotonin and dopamine, are released, aiding in your sleep.
- Use guided meditation in bed. It is helpful to keep headphones by your bed. Make sure that the meditation you listen to is specifically for sleep, as daytime meditations can be stimulating. I love listening to guided meditations for sleep, and then the next thing I know my alarm is going off because it's morning and I don't remember even falling asleep!
- As you establish your transition routine, remember to implement it whenever possible. Writing it down may help. Your body and mind will work well with more structure.

LIFESTYLE MEDICINE SLEEP RX

- Use your bed for sleep and intimacy only
- Establish a regular sleep cycle for bedtime and waking time
- Minimize bedroom noise and lights
- Increase daytime exposure to sunlight, especially outdoors
- Increase daytime physical activity
- Eliminate nighttime caffeinated beverages
- Limit daytime caffeinated beverages
- Avoid alcohol three hours before bed
- Eliminate after-dinner and late-night snacking
- Avoid high-sodium foods, which block vasodilation
- Increase daytime hydration, especially in the late afternoon, to increase vasodilation
- Avoid overexertion as pain can disrupt sleep
- Limit work and other stimulating activities 90 minutes before bed
- Create a wind-down transition routine 1 hour before bed and minimize stress:
  - Decrease light 1 hour before bed, especially blue light
  - Increase bedtime peripheral cutaneous vasodilation (stay warm):
    - Take a bath or shower
    - Wear socks
    - Drink warm, noncaffeinated tea or beverages

- Use adequate blankets
- Use a heating pad
- Listen to calming music
- Read a physical book (no blue light screens)
- Calming breathing tools (pages 45, 53, 109)
- Gentle movement such as yoga or qigong
- Guided meditation (page 127)
- Calming scents (candles, soaps, lotions)
- Self-massage
- Gratitude practice or counting wins

If you are like me and many of my physician clients, you may be looking at this list and feeling that you need to do "all the things," which can get overwhelming. Remember the 1% rule: Focus on getting just 1% better today. Consider starting by implementing just 1 or a few of the Sleep Rx items at a time. And then, just like with the other tools, notice how you feel. As you find what tools work best for you, add them to your toolbox to help you sleep better.

TIME TO TRANSFORM!

For a downloadable version of this worksheet, go to StressFreeMD.net/worksheets

BEHAVIOR CHANGE: SLEEP
What sleep-related behavior would you like to change?

Identify your current stage in changing the behavior you identified above and circle your answer:

1. Precontemplation – *You don't believe that you need to change.*

2. Contemplation – *You're thinking about making a change within the next 6 months.*

3. Preparation – *You're aware of the need for change and plan on taking steps within 1 month. During this phase, you may set a goal and write out the steps you need to take.*

4. Action – *You've started making a change but have been doing it for less than 6 months and haven't yet reached your goal.*

5. Maintenance – *You've reached your goal and sustained the desired behavior for over 6 months.*

If you are not at least at stage 3, do the thought work necessary to get there. (Pages 38-42)

On a scale of 1-10, how confident are you that you can make the desired change? Circle your answer.

        1 2 3 4 5 6 7 8 9 10

On a scale of 1-10, how important is it to you to make the change? Circle your answer.

        1 2 3 4 5 6 7 8 9 10

If you scored lower than a 7 for either confidence or importance, do the thought work needed to score higher. (Pages 38-42)

If you scored a 7 or above, you're ready to set your goals.

CALMER GOALS

C: Clear – Be as clear and detailed as possible when describing what you want to achieve.

A: Assessable – You can assess if there has been any change in your behavior using concrete measurements.

L: Limited – Your goal has a limited time frame and scope, including a beginning and end date.

M: Meaningful – The goal is meaningful and applicable to your life and you understand why you want to achieve it.

E: Exciting – You feel excited to achieve your goal and know you can maintain motivation over an extended period of time.

R: Reachable – Your goal is not too much of an ask and is something you know you can really achieve.

What can you do to improve your stress with respect to sleep just 1% today?

5

Stress Less, Move Better

"Move your body, change your mind."

—Rachel Hollis

> **TOOL: PROGRESSIVE MUSCLE RELAXATION**
>
> With this tool, you will alternate sensing the contraction and release of specific muscle groups in your body paired with cleansing breaths.
>
> 1. Find a comfortable seated or lying-down position. Remove your socks and shoes if you would like and if seated, feel your feet touching the ground. Soften or close your eyes if that feels okay for you.
> 2. **Right lower extremity**: Inhale through your nose and curl your toes. Flex your foot and tighten all the muscles in your right leg all the way up to your buttock. Sense that. Open your mouth, exhale, and release. Sense that.
> 3. **Left lower extremity**: Inhale through your nose and curl your toes. Flex your foot and tighten all the muscles

in your left leg all the way up to your buttock. Sense that. Open your mouth, exhale, and release. Sense that.

4. **Right upper extremity**: Inhale through your nose and make a fist with your right hand. Flex your wrist and tighten all the muscles in your right arm to your shoulder. Sense that. Open your mouth, exhale, and release. Sense that.

5. **Left upper extremity**: Inhale through your nose and make a fist with your left hand. Flex your wrist and tighten all the muscles in your left arm to your shoulder. Sense that. Open your mouth, exhale, and release. Sense that.

6. **Abdomen**: Inhale through your nose and draw in and tense the muscles in your abdomen. Sense that. Open your mouth, exhale, and release. Sense that.

7. **Neck and shoulders**: Inhale through your nose and lift your shoulders up toward your ears as far as possible. Sense that. Open your mouth, exhale, and release. Sense that.

8. **Forehead**: Inhale through your nose and raise your eyebrows as far as you can. Sense that. Open your mouth, exhale, and release. Sense that.

9. **Eyes**: Inhale through your nose and close your eyes tightly. Sense that. Open your mouth, exhale, and release. Sense that.

10. **Whole body**: Inhale through your nose and tighten your whole body. Sense that. Open your mouth, exhale, and release. Sense that.

11. Pause for a moment and notice how you are feeling.
12. Fill out your worksheet for this tool. (StressFreeMD.net/worksheets)
13. If you enjoyed this tool, add it to your toolbox. (Page 35)

Progressive Muscle Relaxation Video

RUNNING FROM THE TIGER

When your mind and body think there is an emergency happening (real or imaginary), your sympathetic nervous system is activated and preps you for that emergency. One way it does that is by increasing muscular tension in your body and taking "the stance": standing with your feet apart, knees slightly bent, hunched forward, shoulders lifted upward, elbows bent, fingers spread, as if you are gearing up to run away from a wild tiger. For me, this is analogous to running away from myself, Dr. Tiger, because my stressful thoughts were like my own volatile internal tiger, chasing me and elevating my chronic stress to extreme levels.

Most of the time when you feel stress, there is no actual wild tiger. There is only a thought that sets up a cascade of events in your body. And over time with chronic stress, your brain believes this is the "new norm," and your body gets stuck in this uncomfortable shape with shortened, tense muscles that remain contracted 24/7. I call this "Tin Man syndrome," like the Tin Man from *The Wizard of Oz*, trapped in your immobile body.

POSTURE EXPERIENTIAL: THE LIMITS OF STRETCHING

Try this:

1. Sit up tall and stretch your shoulders back.
2. Then relax to how you were before.
3. Sit up tall and stretch your shoulders back.
4. Then relax to how you were before.
5. Sit up tall and stretch your shoulders back.
6. Then relax to how you were before.

What did you notice?

When your muscles are tight, you try to stretch and stretch, but it only feels good temporarily because as soon as you release the stretch, what did you notice happened? Your body went right back to where you started. Each time you sat up tall and stretched your shoulders back, you felt good temporarily but then, once released, you resumed the tenser, more hunched state, right?

So what did you just learn? Stretching may feel good temporarily but it doesn't have lasting effects.

Why? Because stretching is *only* a spinal cord reflex and doesn't involve your brain.

Posture Experiential Video

TOOL: RELEASE THE TIN MAN

Now try this somatics-based exercise instead:

1. Find a comfortable seated position. Remove your socks and shoes if you would like and feel your feet touching the ground. Soften or close your eyes if that feels okay for you.
2. Comfortably turn your head to the right and remember what you see—this position is your neutral right.
3. Comfortably turn your head to the left and remember what you see—this position is your neutral left.
4. Turn your head back to your neutral right.
5. Tip your head toward your left shoulder and lift your left shoulder. Sense the contraction. Slowly release your shoulder back down completely, sensing it as you bring your head back to neutral right. Repeat this 3-5 times.
6. Turn your head to your neutral left.
7. Tip your head toward your right shoulder and lift your right shoulder. Sense the contraction. Slowly release your shoulder back down completely, sensing it as you bring your head back to neutral left. Repeat this 3-5 times.
8. Turn your head to center.
9. Tip your head toward your right shoulder. Lift your right shoulder. Tip your head back. Sense the contractions. Then slowly lower your right shoulder completely, sensing that as you bring your head back to center. Repeat 3-5 times.

10. Tip your head toward your left shoulder. Lift your left shoulder. Tip your head back. Sense the contractions. Then slowly lower your left shoulder completely, sensing that as you bring your head back to center. Repeat 3-5 times.

11. Turn your head comfortably to your neutral right. How far can you turn your head now? What do your eyes see?

12. Turn your head comfortably to your neutral left. How far can you turn your head now? What do your eyes see?

13. Pause for a moment and notice how you are feeling.

14. Fill out your worksheet for this tool. (StressFreeMD.net/worksheets)

15. If you enjoyed this tool, add it to your toolbox. (Page 35) (Do it the next day if using it for sleep).

Somatic Neck and Shoulder Release Video

PRINCIPLES OF SOMATICS

Did this work better for you than stretching? Did you increase the range of motion (ROM) in your neck and shoulders? Do you no longer feel like the Tin Man?

This form of movement, the opposite of stretching, called somatic yoga (or what I nicknamed simply "somatics") was taught to me by my octogenarian mentors and has totally changed my life and the lives of thousands of my clients. I get lots of *ooohs* and *aaaahs* with this one!

Now I don't want you to see the word yoga and run the other way. This is not yoga full of spandex and upside-down, twisty shapes. As you just experienced, it's a very therapeutic, comfortable, scientific, and specific way of movement that is based on 2 key components:

1. **Pandiculation**: contracting into chronically tight muscles (also called eccentric contraction) and slowly releasing contractions. This is the opposite of stretching muscles.

2. **Interoception**: sensing the movements, contractions, and de-contractions or relaxation of your muscles. This movement, unlike stretching, is more than a spinal cord reflex because it engages your brain and allows for brain reeducation, reminding your brain of your normal (not chronically contracted) muscle length.

Pandiculation and interoception work together to increase the resting length of your chronically tight muscles so you can feel more spacious and comfortable in your body.

The Tin Man needs oil to release his movement. You need nothing external to yourself to utilize the concepts of somatics. Once you go back to your anatomy and identify which muscles are tight, you can apply these concepts and find lasting relief all by yourself.

SOMATICS STORIES

Somatics has been incredibly life-changing for me as well as for so many of my clients. Let me share a few transformational stories.

My Story

Several years ago, I was in a frightening multivehicle car accident. A driver coming from a crossroad to my left ran a stop sign and cut directly in front of me. I had no stop sign and nowhere to go on the narrow road except into the right side of that car. A third car coming in the opposite direction to me hit the left side of that car as well. Luckily, although all of the cars were no longer drivable and needed to be towed, everybody walked away.

Within the first week following the accident, I started developing progressive neck, shoulder, and jaw pain from delayed onset whiplash. I spent years visiting physiatrists, chiropractors, physical therapists, massage therapists, and acupuncturists and taking several different types of medications without relief. I felt terrible every day, with my right shoulder stuck in a higher and more forward position than my left. It wasn't until I learned somatics, many years later, that I was finally able to relieve all that chronic tension by myself. My shoulders evened out, I felt amazing, and I no longer needed any other treatments or medications. It was magical!

My Clients' Stories

One of my regular yoga therapy clients booked 5 private sessions with me for her 80-year-old husband as a holiday gift. I had never met him before. While I was peering outside the studio room awaiting his arrival, I saw an older gentleman walking toward the studio completely hunched over, short of breath, leaning on his cane, and moving extremely slowly. I didn't realize he was my new client until he entered the studio.

I immediately got him seated and did a quick intake to learn about his complex medical history and how I could best support him. I began by teaching him somatic-based movements to open his chest, back, and shoulders in addition to some plantar fascia work. At the end of the first session, he was sitting up in his chair with improved posture and breathing much more comfortably.

To my surprise, he got out of the chair without my help, posture upright, the cane in his hand barely touching the floor with each step he took. He turned to look back to me and said, "Thanks, Doc, I haven't felt this good in years!" As he walked out of the room, I sat there in awe. I was blown away. That was the first dramatic transformation I'd seen right in front of my eyes based on a single session.

I also witnessed multiple incredible transformations during one of my research studies. I was asked to develop a somatic-based yoga and meditation protocol for individuals suffering from symptoms from chemotherapy-induced peripheral neuropathy (CIPN), an unfortunately common side effect that is usually not relieved with medications. Symptoms include pain, numbness, and tingling in their hands and feet. Over the years, I heard time and time again from patients who participated in my classes how much better they felt but until my studies were published, there had been no documented data.

One of my research participants, a gentleman in his 40s with a history of colon cancer, was distraught over his inability to button his own dress shirt due to the terrible neuropathy in his hands. His dress shirt would get soaked with sweat every morning as he tried to button it, and he would then need to change his shirt and have his wife button it for him. He felt helpless and frustrated. On the last day of the research series, he told me with tears in his eyes that he was able to finally button his own shirt again and thanked me for saving his life. I got teary as well and told him to thank himself for the courage to participate in our study and for learning how to heal himself.

In that same research study, a woman in her 60s with a history of breast cancer described her neuropathy, which caused such pain and numbness in her hands and feet that she could not balance on one foot or hold a washcloth in her hand to wash her feet in the shower. Instead, she had to wash her feet by putting the washcloth on the floor of the shower and standing on it to wipe her feet. After the research series, she gave me a huge hug and shared that she was once again able to balance on one foot and hold the washcloth in her hand while washing the other foot. Her tears were flowing while sharing her transformation and again, I had to hold back mine.

In a class I teach for military veterans, one of my clients in his 70s described suffering from chronic back pain. He had severe PTSD, and the one thing that he loved to do was to garden, but he could only garden for about an hour at a time before the pain set in. After learning somatics, he showed up to class one day with a big smile on his face, sharing that he was now able to garden for 5 hours at a time without pain (and he brought me a bouquet of flowers from his garden).

These are just a few of the incredibly amazing transformations that I have personally experienced and have had the privilege to witness as my clients learn to incorporate somatics into their lives. It's become an imperative part of my daily self-care routine and I highly encourage you to try it. You can find out more about my somatic-based programs on page 213.

OUT OF BREATH

Somatics is a wonderful type of movement to release chronic tension from your body. It is so mindful and calming. Longer relaxed muscles can then be strengthened through cardiovascular and functional fitness, but that is quite difficult to do when you easily run out of breath.

When I moved from flat New Jersey to mountainous North Carolina, I could barely catch my breath, simply walking with my dog up my driveway or keeping up while hiking with our neighbors in their 70s, who were incredibly fit. I was out of breath, and they seemed to float over the hills. At first, I thought I was just adjusting to the altitude difference, but after a few weeks, it was clear that was not the case.

Initially, I thought I just needed to add more cardiovascular exercise to my workouts, so I began taking more cardiovascular-focused classes in an effort to increase my aerobic capacity. I didn't have a plan—I just went to class thinking I was doing enough. It wasn't until I started studying Lifestyle Medicine that I learned the medical literature defines very specific weekly exercise criteria the average adult needs in both quantity and intensity of cardiovascular exercise. In all my years as a gym rat, I never knew this:

> The American College of Sports Medicine and the CDC recommend that adults get a minimum of 150 minutes of moderate intensity exercise per week, or 75 minutes of vigorous exercise per week, as well as muscle-strengthening activities twice a week that work all major muscle groups.

I was already fulfilling the weekly muscle strengthening criteria with the other fitness classes I was taking, but I was not even close to the cardiovascular criteria! If you are like me, you may easily conceptualize the quantity criteria by measuring the number of exercise minutes. But what about *intensity*? It's a bit like a recipe, and the main ingredient I was missing was intensity. It's one that I have found so many other people are missing as well because they don't know about it. Did you?

This was a totally new concept to me: there are 3 levels of exercise intensity.

> While you can determine the 3 levels by measuring your heart rate, an easier way to test the level of intensity is to do the "talk-sing test" and see if you can talk and/or sing while you exercise:
>
> **Mild**: Mild exercise raises your heart rate by a maximum of 63%. While doing mild exercise, you're able to both talk and sing.
>
> **Moderate**: Moderate exercise raises your heart rate by 64-76%. During moderate exercise, you can talk but are not able to sing.
>
> **Vigorous**: Vigorous exercise increases your heart rate by 77-100%. During vigorous exercise, you cannot talk or sing.

Learning these recommendations totally changed how I thought about exercise. When I changed my routine to alternate the appropriate aerobic and strength training combination, my performance drastically improved. I have far surpassed walking up my driveway and can hike to high peaks in a single bound—well, not exactly, but I feel much closer to a superhero now for sure. I really do feel amazing, and many of my clients have similar stories as they've changed how they exercise to match these recommendations and have improved the quality of their lives. Some do say they feel like superheroes!

EXERCISE FOR YOUR BODY AND MIND

Does exercise feel like just one more thing you have to do? Besides achieving that superhero feeling, let's look at why it is so beneficial for your body and mind on a scientific level.

Extensive medical research shows that exercise decreases stress and anxiety and elevates your mood. Physical activity is associated with improved physical health, life satisfaction, cognitive functioning, and psychological well-being. Conversely, physical inactivity is associated with the development of psychological disorders, including Alzheimer's dementia. Yes, even dementia. Scary, right?

Exercise also makes you feel good because it increases dopamine, serotonin, and endorphin levels. The ripple effect is that your mood is elevated when you exercise, so you feel better about yourself—you have more self-esteem and confidence, and as you're getting stronger and your body feels better, you also begin to look better and your clothes fit better, which only increases your self-confidence even more.

BENEFITS OF EXERCISE

Exercise benefits us in many ways:

- **Improves sleep quality**: Exercise improves the quality of your sleep, though it's important to exercise earlier in the day because it heats up the body and can make it difficult for your core to cool, which is necessary for sleep. (For more information on sleep, see chapter 4.)

- **Decreases anxiety and depression**: Exercise is an anti-depressive and an anxiolytic (has an anti-anxiety effect). Cognitive behavioral therapy has been found to be as effective as medication in treating depression, and exercise is comparable to cognitive behavioral therapy in treating depression.[41]

- **Reduces blood pressure**: Exercise keeps blood flowing properly, supplying oxygen and nutrients, removing waste, and preventing serious health conditions such as heart attacks and strokes.

- **Lowers risk of heart disease, stroke, and type 2 diabetes**: Exercise lowers the risk of the most common diseases in the world: heart disease, stroke, and type 2 diabetes. In fact, an adequate amount of moderate intensity exercise reduces the risk of cardiovascular disease by 20-30%.
- **Lowers risk of certain cancers**: Exercise lowers your risk of certain cancers, particularly breast and colon cancer, which are two of the most common cancers:
  - Reduces primary onset and recurrence of breast cancer.
  - Improves symptoms and quality of life during cancer treatment.
  - Improves survival of cancer.
- **Improves bone health**: Bones strengthen in 2 ways: through compressive forces such as weight training, and tensile forces, which are lengthening exercises such as yoga. In fact, research has shown that people who only do yoga still increase their bone density even if they are not standing and are practicing yoga only on the floor and in chairs.[42]
- **Reduces risk of dementia**: Exercise increases levels of brain-derived neurotropic factor (BDNF), which is like Miracle Gro for your brain—it increases neurogenesis and network connectivity.[43]
- **Controls blood glucose**: Exercise provides adequate energy to cells and vital organs and prevents serious health conditions including diabetes.
- **Controls weight**: Exercise in combination with calorie reduction results in significant and sustainable weight loss.
- **Reduces cholesterol**: Exercise helps to prevent atherosclerotic plaque formation.
- **Increases life expectancy**: People who get the most exercise have the least number of years of life lost, independent of

their weight. Studies of people who were overweight and people who were thin showed that even those who were obese had the least number of years of life lost if they worked out regularly. In this study, obesity wasn't the problem—it was the lack of movement.[44]

- **Improves the gut microbiome**: Progressive increase in physical activity level is associated with increased levels of short-chain fatty acids (SCFA) and bacterial diversity.[45]

YOUR BODY WAS MADE TO MOVE

While exercise has many benefits, lack of activity increases morbidity and mortality and causes the *opposite* of the effects listed above. It actually makes you sick!

Unfortunately, according to Medscape statistics,[46] only 24% of physicians exercise 4-5 times per week, 34% exercise 2-3 times per week, 20% exercise once a week or less, and 10% never exercise.

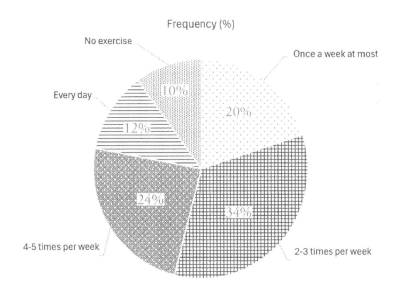

Graphic produced using data from Medscape Physician Lifestyle & Happiness Report 2024: The Ongoing Struggle for Balance, *https://www.medscape.com/slideshow/2024-lifestyle-happiness-6016860#9*

As the gatekeepers of health, physicians are not doing a good job of caring for themselves or setting a good example for their patients.

People in general aren't moving their bodies enough. Only 1 in 3 adults achieves the recommended amount of physical activity per week. This means 66% of Americans are physically inactive. Compare this to 13.7% of the population who smoke cigarettes.[47]

There was a 50% reduction in daily exercise across data for populations in 163 countries from 2000 to 2022, according to a *Lancet* article published in 2024.[48] That's largely due to technology, such as cars, television, and the internet. Our lives have gotten very sedentary, and the medical field, in particular, has become more sedentary, moving from traditional handwritten charts to charting in the EHR (electronic health record) and going from traditional film to filmless in radiology utilizing PACS digital imaging.

Sitting has become the new smoking. In other words, sitting is killing people! Our bodies weren't meant to be sedentary. In fact, 6.9% of all-cause mortality is due to sitting.[49]

You can help avoid prolonged sitting by including at least 5 minutes of movement per hour. If you can, get up from your desk and march in place, do some jumping jacks, push-ups, or squats—not only will it help mitigate the effects of sitting, but it'll also help you feel more alert and focused.

> **Myth**: You can make up for all the time you spend sitting by getting enough exercise.
>
> **Truth**: Exercise doesn't counteract a sedentary lifestyle.

Research shows that people who exercise but still sit in front of the TV for several hours a day still have an increased all-cause mortality equivalent to those who watched TV and never exercised.[50] Harvard reports that excessive sitting is a lethal activity.[51] Whether it's sitting in front of the TV or sitting in front of your computer working, charting, or reading cases, it's way too much sitting! So it's simple: Exercise is really good for you, and sitting is really bad for you. It doesn't balance out.

> **RISKS OF SEDENTARY LIFESTYLE**[52]
> - Hypertension
> - Cardiovascular disease
> - Weight gain/obesity
> - Cancer
> - Osteoporosis
> - Anxiety and depression
> - Stroke
> - Type 2 diabetes

As I spend more time working at my computer, I too have to remind myself to get up and move more. I actually set the alarm on my phone to remind myself each hour to move. What do I do? I have a mat in my office and I do push-ups, sit-ups, and standing squats, and I get some fresh air outside. It's a wonderful reset. I got a standing desk and a small under-desk treadmill so that I can stand more when working and move my body.

How can you become less sedentary in your life?

HOW ARE YOU MOVING?

I invite you to take a moment to do a nonjudgmental movement self-inquiry:

- How many minutes of movement are you getting on a daily and weekly basis?
- Are you doing enough cardio?
- Are you exercising at the right intensity?
- Are you incorporating strength training?
- How sedentary are you?
- Do you need to get up and move more?
- Does tension need to be relieved in your body?
- Do you prefer exercising alone or with others?

What did you learn about yourself?

GET ORGANIZED

Exercise and movement are highly personal. To create a routine that works for you, consider what you enjoy doing, your schedule, and your motivations.

I have found the one thing that has helped me get started the most is getting organized. For example, if you are exercising from home, the night before, lay out your exercise clothing and towel, fill up your water bottle, and set out anything else you may need for easy access. I leave these things on the bench in my bathroom, which is one of the first things I see when I walk in. If you're heading to the gym before work in the morning or right after work, pack up your bag the night before with everything you need for exercising and showering, a snack, water, and workout clothes and put it in your car so you won't forget it in the morning.

Getting organized in these ways helps you not waste time in the morning scrounging around, hurriedly trying to get it all together. It also keeps you accountable with no "I don't have time to get my gym stuff ready" excuses.

If you are taking a group class at a fitness center or online, register ahead of time and set a reminder in your phone calendar. There is something about seeing an activity listed in your calendar that helps hold you accountable. I take some early morning preregistered classes at the gym and I know that the instructor keeps tabs on who is showing up, so I feel much more accountable to show up when I preschedule my workouts at the gym. If working out with others is what you enjoy, find a workout buddy and get those workouts scheduled in your calendars.

Our physician brains don't like to do anything wrong. We have perfectionistic tendencies, which in some cases (like this one) can work to your advantage.

SOMETHING IS BETTER THAN NOTHING

If you are someone who has an all-or-none philosophy, you may think that you don't have time for 150 minutes of moderate-intensity or 75 minutes of vigorous exercise each week, and you may feel overwhelmed by this. What happens when you feel overwhelmed? You end up not doing anything at all. This is a common thought pattern in physicians, who tend to have perfectionistic personalities (ahem, me included) and in this situation, perfectionism works against you.

But here is some key research to offset that thinking. Know that doing something is definitely better than doing nothing. Research shows that just 15 minutes of moderate exercise per day had a 14% reduced risk of all-cause mortality and a 3-year longer life expectancy![53] So even just 15 minutes per day reduces your risk of mortality and extends your life!

I know that setting aside time for exercise may seem impossible, especially when you're exhausted from work and stress. But no matter what your life looks like, I invite you to give yourself the gift of movement for at least 15 minutes per day. When I ask my busiest physician clients what the least amount of time is they have in any given day to care for themselves, the most common lowest number is 15 minutes. Based on the literature, even 15 minutes a day is effective. Remember that your life literally depends on it. Think about anything else you do that takes 15 minutes in your day that you could replace—maybe watching TV or scrolling on social media? We all have at least 15 minutes a day to move our bodies!

If pain is keeping you from exercising, stop playing doctor or putting it off and hoping it will get better. Hope is not a plan. Consider getting evaluated and, if cleared, find adaptive exercises that allow you to work around that pain and move other body parts. I've had multiple injuries and have never stopped exercising. It can even improve pain in some cases and help you build strength to avoid future injuries. And somatic movement is a safe and effective way to relieve pain from chronically tense muscles. There's always a way you can move your body, and any movement is better than nothing. Movement is medicine!

HOW TO ADD MOVEMENT THROUGHOUT THE DAY

Find small ways that you can incorporate more movement into your day. It will make a big difference in how you feel. It will increase your energy level and your ability to focus while decreasing your stress level. Find the kinds of exercise you like and that you'll actually do, then build a routine around those things.

- Use a standing desk or treadmill desk at work.
- Take the stairs over an elevator.
- Park further away in the parking lot to walk to the entrance.
- Bike to work.
- Set a phone alarm to ensure you get up from your chair for at least 5 minutes every hour of sitting. Do push-ups, squats, or jumping jacks, go for a quick walk outside, or do anything that gets you moving.
- Make active social plans. Take an exercise class together, go on a hike with friends, or walk while talking on the phone. Having an exercise buddy can also be a great way to stay accountable.

Movement is medicine.

TIME TO TRANSFORM!

For a downloadable version of this worksheet, go to StressFreeMD.net/worksheets

BEHAVIOR CHANGE: EXERCISE

What exercise-related behavior would you like to change?

Identify your current stage in changing the behavior you identified above and circle your answer:

1. Precontemplation – *You don't believe that you need to change.*

2. Contemplation – *You're thinking about making a change within the next 6 months.*

3. Preparation – *You're aware of the need for change and plan on taking steps within 1 month. During this phase, you may set a goal and write out the steps you need to take.*

4. Action – *You've started making a change but have been doing it for less than 6 months and haven't yet reached your goal.*

5. Maintenance – *You've reached your goal and sustained the desired behavior for over 6 months.*

If you are not at least at stage 3, do the thought work necessary to get there. (Pages 38-42)

On a scale of 1-10, how confident are you that you can make the desired change? Circle your answer.

        1   2   3   4   5   6   7   8   9   10

On a scale of 1-10, how important is it to you to make the change? Circle your answer.

        1   2   3   4   5   6   7   8   9   1

If you scored lower than a 7 for either confidence or importance, do the thought work needed to score higher. (Pages 38-42)

If you scored a 7 or above, you're ready to set your goals.

FITT GOALS

Creating goals around fitness is a little bit different than other types of goals. While the CALMER goal acronym can still be helpful in regard to fitness, there's a more specific acronym that can help you to create effective movement and exercise goals, called FITT.

FITT goals establish 4 key components:

- **Frequency** – How often will you exercise?
- **Intensity** – What intensity level will the exercise be: mild, moderate, or intense?
- **Time** – How many minutes will you perform the exercise?
- **Type** – What type of exercise will you perform?

Frequency: How often will you exercise?

Monday	Tuesday	Wednesday	Thursday	Friday	Saturday	Sunday

Intensity: Mild, moderate, intense, or a combination?

Time: How many minutes will you perform the exercise?

Type: What type of exercise will you perform?

What can you do to improve your stress with respect to exercise just 1% today?

6

Stress Less, Connect Better

"Medicine and technology may fail us at times,
but human connection grounded in love
and compassion always heals."

—Dr. Vivek Murthy, 19th and 21st Surgeon General of the United States, Author of *Together: The Healing Power of Human Connection in a Sometimes Lonely World*

TOOL: THE POWER OF YOUR SMILE

If I asked you, "What makes you smile?" you would think of things that make you feel happy. But what if I told you that it can also happen in the *opposite* direction? Your smile itself can make you feel happy!

1. Find a comfortable seated or lying down position. If you would like, remove your socks and shoes and if sitting, feel your feet touching the ground. Soften or close your eyes if that feels okay for you.
2. Create a smile shape with your mouth by turning the corners of your mouth upward.

3. Hold that smile for a few moments. You can relax your gaze or close your eyes if you would like.
4. Pause for a moment and notice how you are feeling.
5. Fill out your worksheet for this tool. (StressFreeMD.net/worksheets)
6. If you enjoyed this tool, add it to your toolbox. (Page 35)

The Power of Your Smile Video

SMILE ANATOMY AND PHYSIOLOGY

When you smile and turn the corners of your mouth upward, you engage your circular facial muscles. These muscles, innervated by the facial nerve, cranial nerve 7, signal to your brain that you are smiling. Your brain then releases the good feeling hormones dopamine and serotonin as well as endorphins—natural pain killers that boost your mood. Stress hormones (cortisol and catecholamines) are lowered, as is your blood pressure.[54]

As the saying goes, "When you smile, the whole world smiles with you." Smiling not only makes you feel better, but it affects others too. When you smile, you appear more likable, courteous, and confident, and it is contagious (in a good way) as it encourages others to smile back at you. A British study reported that smiling creates the same level of brain stimulation as up to 2,000 chocolate bars or $25,000![55]

SEEING WHAT ISN'T THERE

During the morning conference at the beginning of each academic year, one of my favorite radiology attendings would show the first-year residents a chest x-ray. One by one, he would call them up to review the case, and one by one, each resident was unable to identify the finding. He would then move on to calling on one of the second-years who remembered being in the hot seat the year before and quickly gave the correct answer. So are you curious? What was the finding? The answer is this: cleidocranial dysostosis, absent clavicles (collarbones).

I learned early during my training that when evaluating an imaging study, it is so much easier to identify a present abnormality, such as a measurable lesion that you can see on an image, than it is to identify something that is missing. It is hard to see what *isn't* there. I have found this to be true not only when reading out imaging studies but also in everyday life.

IF I ONLY HAD A HEART

For much of my career as a diagnostic radiologist, like many healthcare professionals suffering from chronic stress and burnout, just getting through the day felt robotic and at times numb. Making time to connect with others wasn't even listed on the to-do checklist when you are living inside this busy isolating bubble, extremely focused on just surviving each workday. And then this robotic tendency leaves with you when you exit the hospital or office and spills over into your life outside of work.

I experienced a significant shift away from this bubble when I began implementing stress-relief tools. I remember thinking that it felt as if I was in *The Wizard of Oz*, where everything had been black and white and it suddenly turned to color. I was like the Scarecrow who suddenly got a heart and could finally feel—actually feel! I'll never forget that impactful moment I shared with you earlier in this book about transitioning to "eyes open," when my then very young daughter said to me, "Mommy, I love it when you look at me in my eyes when I'm talking to you, Mommy."

What shifted in me? Presence. I became so much more present that even my young child noticed. I had no idea what I was lacking until she helped me to see what wasn't there, both in my own life and in the lives of the people I cared about. Presence is a present, a gift, and is necessary for a key component to health and well-being: connection.

LESSONS FROM THE SOUTH

While living in the hustle and bustle of the Northeast, I used to play a little game with my young kids when traveling through the airport. I would say, "Let's see who can be the first one to identify someone who makes eye contact, smiles, or says hello. Ready, set, go!" And guess what would happen: there was no winner. We would get through the entire airport and, sadly, neither of my kids would be able to identify anyone who did any of those things. Now, living in the South, things are quite different. From the moment you step into the airport, you can feel a lightness. People are genuinely courteous, making eye contact, smiling, and saying hi. My husband and I relocated while empty-nesting and our adult children haven't had a chance to play that game here. But what I do know is that if we did play it, someone would definitely be a quick winner!

While practicing medicine in the Northeast, I used to be able to leave the hospital after work and within 20 to 30 minutes, I could run several quick errands including the dry cleaner, the pharmacy, the bank, the supermarket, the post office, and finally home. Here, in the South, I can't run all those errands so quickly because strangers stop me, look me in the eyes and ask, "How are you?" And they *really* want to know! And even though I may now only be able to get one errand done in 30 minutes, I've come to love and embrace that connectivity.

What I have learned is that people in the South seem to understand and prioritize the importance of social connection. It is not something we often think about in a medical sense, but it may surprise you that there is plenty of research showing that it's extremely important for your health and well-being.

Your positive social connections with others positively affect your autonomic nervous system. When you're socially connected, you activate your parasympathetic nervous system and relaxation response, which decreases cortisol, lowers your heart rate and blood pressure, decreases inflammation associated with chronic disease, and ultimately increases your longevity.

Positive social connections also increase the hormone oxytocin, the bonding and love hormone, which improves your overall mental and emotional well-being. This results in an increase in your sense of belonging and purpose.

The saying goes, "The purpose of life is to live a life of purpose." I like to add, "and to live life *on purpose.*" When you are intentionally making social connections that feed your greatest good, you are living your life *on purpose* and elevating your own health and well-being.

On the flip side, lack of social connection, social isolation, and loneliness can be extremely damaging. It increases the risk of heart disease, hypertension, diabetes, dementia, and depression. Lacking connection can increase the risk of premature death to levels comparable to smoking daily!

As a Diagnostic Radiologist, I was particularly blown away when I learned this: Functional MRI research, which allows you to see how certain parts of the brain work in certain situations, identifies that the portion of the brain that is "turned on" during social isolation, the anterior insular cortex, is the same part of the brain that is "turned on" when experiencing physical pain. Your emotions are deeply connected with the pain you feel in your body. The pain of isolation is very real. So now you can understand through the medical literature why social isolation can feel so very painful.[56] Have you ever felt lonely even though you were surrounded by other people? To feel socially connected, you need to have a positive experience with the people you're around. A negative experience only increases the sense of isolation. Social connection is about more than just seeing others—it's about being with people who lift you up, support you, and nourish you.

A study from Harvard showed that the single most important predictor of happiness and longevity is having social connections.[57]

THE LONELINESS EPIDEMIC

For Dr. Vivek Murthy, the U.S. Surgeon General, the levels of loneliness and isolation in our country are of high concern. *The U.S. Surgeon General's Advisory on the Healing Effects of Social Connection and Community*[58] outlines the importance of social connection on our health and the risks of isolation, which is at epidemic levels with about half of adults in the U.S. reporting feelings of loneliness.

Doctors often think that they're here to serve and not to socialize. That sense of serving can become your identity and make you believe you don't deserve to take time to be with others.

Dr. Murthy shared about his own story with social isolation when he was in his first surgeon generalship under President Obama. At the time, he threw himself completely into his work and blocked off the rest of the world. When he was let go after the next election, he realized that for 4 years he hadn't been with his friends or family, and he felt so alone. His wife, Dr. Alice Chen, encouraged him to add connection into his life because she realized he was suffering from loneliness.

After helping himself and during his second term as the U.S. Surgeon General, Dr. Murthy focused on addressing the loneliness epidemic our country has been facing because it's a serious threat to everyone's health.

Social Isolation

Here are some of the effects social isolation has on your well-being:

- Worsens depression
- Increases feelings of lack of self-worth
- Decreases immune function
- Increases inflammation
- Causes poor sleep patterns
- Increases cortisol (stress hormone) levels
- Increases the risk of chronic diseases such as hypertension, coronary artery disease, anxiety, and depression
- Increases risk of premature mortality by 29%

Social Connection

The benefits of social connection go beyond simply reversing the effects of social isolation:

- Increases the level of oxytocin, the love and bonding hormone
- Increases serotonin and dopamine, which are natural antidepressants
- Enhances trust and decreases fear
- Increases eye contact, making you more likely to engage with others
- Increases ability to sense and connect emotionally by picking up on verbal and nonverbal cues, so you feel more present and it's easier to make connections
- Increases empathy
- Activates the parasympathetic nervous system, which improves emotional well-being by reducing stress
- Decreases heart rate
- Improves overall health
- Increases longevity
- Increases a sense of belonging and cultivates purpose
- Alleviates trauma

> "Social connection is as fundamental to our mental and physical health as food, water, and sleep."
>
> —Dr. Vivek Murthy, U.S. Surgeon General

STRESS AND SOCIAL CONNECTION

Have you been tempted to skip out on a social event because you were just too stressed to socialize, but ended up feeling so much better after you went? I know I sure have! That's because connecting with others helps reduce stress.

Social connection, like each of the pillars of Lifestyle Medicine, works bidirectionally with stress. You feel better when you're around other people, and it becomes easier to connect. When you feel less stressed, you become more socially connected.

In contrast, stress can make it more difficult to connect with others. You're more likely to be reactive and say or do things you wish you could take back. Stress also makes it more difficult to sense the feelings and needs of others, increasing that lack of connection.

We've all experienced social isolation at some point during our lives. Just think back to the isolating effects of the pandemic, beginning in March of 2020 when the world shut down. Unfortunately, even prior to the pandemic, social isolation was on the rise as people spend more and more time alone and less time with friends, family, and co-workers. The lives of Americans have become more socially isolating as we move toward working from home and spending much of our time online. Not surprisingly, social isolation also increases as the number of working hours increases.[59]

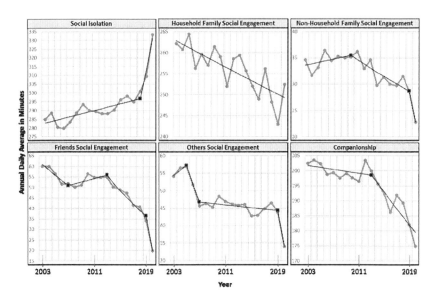

U.S. social connectedness trends, 2003-2020. Annual daily average in minutes are plotted on the thick gray line, representing all age groups, income levels, and race/ethnicity.[60] Joinpoint trendlines (thinner black lines) show inflection points where trends changed.
https://www.ncbi.nlm.nih.gov/pmc/articles/PMC9811250/

I've heard countless stories from my clients whose levels of social connection have significantly improved after implementing tools to reduce their stress. Let me share a few of their amazing comments:

- "You saved my marriage."
- "My staff loves being around me again."
- "I have been getting all of these gifts from my patients."
- "I have become so popular that I can no longer take any new patients."
- "My kids now think I am a cool mom and want to hang out with me."

The quality of your life skyrockets when you are socially connecting in meaningful ways!

THE BLUE ZONES: SOCIAL CONNECTION AND LONGEVITY

Have you ever heard of the amazing blue zones? Blue zones represent specific cities around the world that have the highest number of centenarians (people over 100 years old) who live the longest and healthiest lives. They include Ikaria, Greece; Okinawa, Japan; Sardinia, Italy; Loma Linda, California; and Nicoya, Costa Rica.

Sardinia, Italy, is home to the world's longest-lived men. Okinawa, Japan, is home to the world's longest-lived women. Loma Linda, California, has a Seventh Day Adventist community that outlives the average American by a decade. Ikaria, Greece, is a tiny island community with significantly reduced rates of chronic illness. And in Nicoya, Costa Rica, people are more than twice as likely as Americans to reach 90 years of age.

Each of these blue zones has a number of common cultural behaviors that have been correlated to better health and longevity. These are the 9 behaviors:

1. Getting regular movement throughout the day
2. Having a sense of purpose for your life
3. Prioritizing stress relief
4. Eating until you're about 80% full
5. Eating a plant-based diet
6. Drinking alcohol in moderation
7. Connecting with your community
8. Prioritizing family (biological or chosen)
9. Choosing supportive social circles

Notice that the last 3 on that list are all about improving social connection, and the rest overlap with the pillars of Lifestyle Medicine in one way or another. The blue zones' cultures support healthy lifestyle behaviors, highly prioritizing social connection, which significantly increases the health and longevity of the population.

My First Visit to the Blue Zones

My bucket list includes visiting all of the blue zones to learn and experience firsthand how they live their lives. In 2024, I visited Sardinia, Italy, with my family, and had the privilege of spending an afternoon in the home of a family who live in the blue zone region. The family members who were present during my visit included a 97-year-old woman, her 2 daughters, and her granddaughter. What was my greatest takeaway? Above all else it was their deep connection with one another, which was palpable. The 97-year-old woman was so bright and witty! She had us all laughing, and she invited us to her 100th birthday party in a few years! I am celebrating all that she taught me about the importance of connection.

SOCIAL CONNECTION FOR PHYSICIANS

For physicians, feelings of isolation pose a particular problem. Many feel they are too busy and burned out to cultivate strong social lives, and it can be difficult for people outside of healthcare to relate to the unique experiences of the physician.

The COVID pandemic was a major isolating event for many, but even more so for physicians, especially with respect to their families—many couldn't even sleep in their own beds or homes. Some slept on a different floor from their family members or stayed at long-term rentals. Some just lived at the hospital. Many didn't see their families for weeks or months. They were terrified to bring the virus home and carry that heavy burden of being responsible for infecting their loved ones.

Even without the effects of the COVID pandemic, practicing medicine can be extremely isolating. Shared physician experiences are invaluable in developing social connection, which is why it's often easiest as a physician to make friends with people at your workplace who understand you at a level that others cannot comprehend.

For physicians, it can be difficult to make and keep nonphysician friends and partners because they just don't understand what you have been through and are currently experiencing. I completely understand if a physician friend or client has to cancel their plans with me last-minute, and I don't take offense. We don't punch a clock—and our schedules can change in any moment. It's what we signed up for and there is an unwritten mutual understanding between us. But the rest of the world didn't sign up for it.

This is why 45% of physicians are married to other physicians or healthcare professionals—it makes it so much easier.[61]

Additionally, physician moms often feel very isolated because there's a cultural expectation about how you're going to take care of your family. It was hard for me, being a physician mom in a town with a lot of moms who didn't work at all. I would hear the other moms make negative comments about me under their breath, judging the lifestyle that I chose.

I remember the days I would pick up my then-young children at summer camp and one stay-at-home mom would always hold her son and say while looking at me, "I could never leave him with someone else." I wasn't like the other moms, and they let me know it. And how interesting—when one of their kids got sick or injured, who was the first person that they would call for help to get them into a specialist or review their imaging studies? Me. Then the white coat was acceptable. I learned early on that it is important in these types of situations to recognize that it is not your job to live up to other people's expectations of you—it is your job to just live up to yourself. You do you.

CRAVING CONNECTION: LESSONS FROM MY STUDENTS

Humans crave social connection. "I love feeling lonely," said no one ever. I learned an important lesson from my own students when their sense of connection was abruptly taken away.

I have spent many years diagnosing cancer and wanted to help support my patients at a greater level. Since 2010, I have been volunteering and teaching weekly yoga and meditation classes for cancer recovery. I discovered part of what my students loved was not just what I was teaching them but the connections they were making with each other. They would come early to the studio to meet together before class and then stay after class to spend time with one another. They cultivated special friendships through my class and would email and text each other throughout the week.

After COVID hit and everything shut down, including the yoga studio where I taught these classes, I knew I needed to do something to continue to create this healing space of connection. I remember it clearly. In March 2020, while in the airport flying home from Mexico on a Saturday, I converted my classes to the virtual format. I watched YouTube videos on how to use this thing called Zoom and was ready to teach online by the time we had our next scheduled class that very Monday. When I saw that my computer screen was full, I was teary and felt grateful for this technology.

Following our first few online sessions, many of my students reached out to tell me how happy they were that we were able to continue to have our sessions but also how lonely they felt and how they missed spending time together before and after class. To continue to cultivate that in the virtual space, I decided to open the classes up early and leave class open afterward so they could talk for as long as they liked. This relieved their feelings of being alone and isolated at a time when our whole world had shut down. I could hear them talking for hours after class was over.

With so many people suffering from isolation, I opened those classes up to all. We had people joining from many countries around the world including France, Italy, Ireland, and England, and even had active-duty U.S. Marines joining from Asia!

Here was the biggest lesson: people just need people. Whether you are a physician, someone on the cancer journey, a member of our military, or anyone else, you're born with a need for human connection. It's not just a luxury but truly a necessity for your well-being.

HOW TO IMPROVE YOUR SOCIAL CONNECTIONS

Start by improving your existing relationships. Then you can expand to building new relationships.

Existing Relationships

Schedule connections, no matter how small – Schedule communications and connections, just like I encourage you to do with your other Lifestyle Medicine pillars like fitness or sleep. If something isn't scheduled, you know that it most likely won't happen. Even if you just plan to talk on the phone with a friend or relative while driving home from work, put it on your schedule. Schedule a call, an activity, or even just a text. Put in a reminder to reach out to someone because if you don't, you're going to forget. Reminding yourself to connect even in small ways, like sending a picture, a snapchat, or an emoji, will keep communications open with that individual. Make connecting a priority.

Say yes – Say yes to get-togethers. This is something I've been working on for years. When people invite me to do things, I tend to think I'm too busy, but now I try to say yes as often as I can because finding time to spend with others is so important for your well-being. Have lunch, go for a walk, or go to a friend's house for dinner. When you say yes more often, you'll be happier and more relaxed. The work will still be there when you get back, and you'll have better focus and concentration so you can get things done more quickly than if you hadn't spent the time connecting with others.

New Relationships

Find people like you – Find people you have things in common with. That's likely to be other medical professionals, but it might also be people with other shared interests or hobbies. If you can't find people to connect with, you can try tools like Meetup.com where you can find groups who do all sorts of things. Look for community groups or clubs of people who like to do the same things you do, whether that's hiking, biking, or whatever. Volunteer for an organization you're passionate about and meet people with the same passion.

Permission to Complete

Allow yourself to complete relationships – Connect with people who serve your greatest good and allow yourself to "complete" relationships with those who don't. I like the term "completing" better than saying breaking up with someone or cutting someone out. You change over time, and social connections can be either nourishing or damaging. It's okay to complete relationships that don't serve you. Of course, you may not be able to complete relationships with family members, but outside of that, recognize which social connections are good for you and disengage with the ones that are harming you.

Fitting in Versus Belonging

Focus on the feeling of belonging – Don't worry about fitting in. Instead, focus on finding the feeling of belonging. When I was growing up, curly hair was very unpopular. I remember when feathered hair was in fashion, like Farrah Fawcett from *Charlie's Angels*, and I would blow-dry my hair for nearly an hour each morning to try to look like her (as did everyone else). My hair looked awful and was dry and breaking as a result. But I wanted to fit in and look like everybody else.

This changed one day in college. I was taking a marine biology course in Bermuda where we had morning lectures followed by snorkeling to identify what we had learned. We'd be in the water, then back on the boat, then in the water again, and as my hair dried on the boat, one of my classmates said, "Look at Robyn's hair!" I thought, *Oh no!* and I remember covering my hair with my hands. But then the next comment was, "You should leave it like that. It looks so great! Just be you!" I was shocked. My whole life I'd thought I'd needed to fit in by masking my curls.

I think about that frequently when I think about fitting in versus belonging. People try so hard to fit in and to be like everyone else. Good social connection doesn't come from fitting in—it comes from a sense of belonging. Belonging means showing up as your authentic self and the people you're with loving and accepting you just the way you are.

Being in a group because you're trying to be just like them is not social connection. It's an important distinction: Do you really like the people you're around? Are you trying to be like others just because you want to be around people? That's not nourishing for you. You need to "let your hair be curly" rather than worrying what other people will think.

Live by the words of Mr. Rogers from the children's program *Mr. Roger's Neighborhood*: "I like you just the way you are."

Surround yourself with people who nourish you and lift you up, because in the end, as Ram Dass said, "We are all just walking each other home."

> **TOOL: LOVING KINDNESS MEDITATION**
>
> 1. Find a comfortable seated or lying-down position. Remove your socks and shoes if possible and if seated, feel your feet touching the ground. Soften or close your eyes if that feels okay for you.
> 2. Place your right hand over the center of your chest below your clavicles (collarbones).
> 3. Place your left hand on top of your right hand.
> 4. Take a moment to feel the weight of your hands resting on your body. Feel your hands touching one another.
> 5. Bring to mind an acquaintance, someone you know but not well.

6. Repeat after me quietly or aloud:
   - "May you be happy."
   - "May you be healthy."
   - "May you love and be loved."
   - "May you live your life with ease."
7. Think of someone you love and care about deeply.
8. Repeat after me quietly or aloud:
   - "May you be happy."
   - "May you be healthy."
   - "May you love and be loved."
   - "May you live your life with ease."
9. Think of yourself.
10. Repeat after me quietly or aloud:
    - "May I be happy."
    - "May I be healthy."
    - "May I love and be loved."
    - "May I live my life with ease."
11. Pause for a moment and notice how you are feeling after offering others and yourself loving kindness.
12. Fill out your worksheet for this tool. (StressFreeMD.net/worksheets)
13. If you enjoyed this tool, add it to your toolbox. (Page 35)

Loving Kindness Meditation Video

TIME TO TRANSFORM!

For a downloadable version of this worksheet, go to StressFreeMD.net/worksheets

BEHAVIOR CHANGE: CONNECTION

What behavior related to social connection would you like to change?

Identify your current stage in changing the behavior you identified above:

1. Precontemplation – *You don't believe that you need to change.*

2. Contemplation – *You're thinking about making a change within the next 6 months.*

3. Preparation – *You're aware of the need for change and plan on taking steps within 1 month. During this phase, you may set a goal and write out the steps you need to take.*

4. Action – *You've started making a change but have been doing it for less than 6 months and haven't yet reached your goal.*

5. Maintenance – *You've reached your goal and have sustained the desired behavior for more than 6 months.*

If you are not at least at stage 3, do the thought work necessary to get there. (Pages 38-42)

On a scale of 1-10, how confident are you that you can make the desired change?

1   2   3   4   5   6   7   8   9   10

On a scale of 1-10, how important is it to you to make the change?

1   2   3   4   5   6   7   8   9   10

If you scored lower than a 7 for either confidence or importance, do the thought work needed to score higher. (Pages 38-42)

If you scored a 7 or above, you're ready to set some goals.

CALMER GOALS

C: Clear – Be as clear and detailed as possible when describing what you want to achieve.

A: Assessable – You can assess if there has been any change in your behavior using concrete measurements.

L: Limited – Your goal has a limited time frame and scope, including a beginning and end date.

M: Meaningful – The goal is meaningful and applicable to your life and you understand why you want to achieve it.

E: Exciting – You feel excited to achieve your goal and know you can maintain motivation over an extended period of time.

R: Reachable – Your goal is not too much of an ask and is something you know you can really achieve.

What can you do to improve your stress with respect to connection by just 1% today?

7

Stress Less, Say "No" Better

"Yesterday I was clever so I wanted to change the world. Today I am wise so I'm changing myself."

—Rumi

TOOL: WHAT'S GOING RIGHT?

Your brain is filled with at least 60,000 thoughts per day. Have you ever noticed how many of them are negative? Have you noticed that you are having an internal conversation all day long with even more negative thoughts?

That's your default network always looking for and pointing out what is going wrong in your life. It can weigh you down and make you feel pretty awful, leading you to make unhealthy choices that you often regret later—bringing on more negative self-talk.

I invite you to turn those negative thoughts around and try this tool I personally find very helpful, and I use at the beginning of all of my coaching client sessions. I call it "What's Going Right?"

1. Get a piece of paper and a pen or open a blank note on your phone or computer.
2. Find a comfortable seated position.
3. Ask yourself this question: "What's going right?" *Nothing is too small.* It could simply be "Someone smiled at me and held the door for me. I felt the warm sun on my face. I woke up today. My tea smells amazing."
4. Write down all your answers.
5. Ask yourself the question again, and write down some more, until you have run out of answers.
6. Read back your answers aloud, if you're able to, or read them quietly if need be.
7. If you'd like, record your answers and play them back and listen.
8. Celebrate your wins and all that *is* going right in your life!
9. Pause for a few moments and notice how you feel.
10. Fill out your worksheet for this tool. (StressFreeMD.net/worksheets)
11. If you enjoyed this tool, add it to your toolbox. (Page 35)

What's Going Right Video

UNHEALTHY HABITS

So far, I've covered stress as it relates to the Lifestyle Medicine pillars of nutrition, sleep, exercise, and social connection. Next up is the pillar of avoiding risky substances. But I'm approaching this chapter a little bit differently. This chapter is not *just* about saying no to risky substances—I have found this pillar to be much broader and extensive. It's really about saying no to many types of unhealthy habits beyond risky substance use. What do I mean by unhealthy habits? Unhealthy habits include any escape you use to steer clear of your unwanted stressful feelings and emotions.

Feelings Versus Emotions

What's the difference between a feeling and an emotion? The terms are frequently used interchangeably, but there is a difference: a feeling is the *somatic expression* of an emotion. It's what you sense in your body when an emotion is present.

For example, if your emotion is anger, how do you know anger is there? You know its associated sensations in your body, which may include feeling hot, sweaty, tense, or you may experience palpitations. If your emotion is sadness, how do you know sadness is there? You know because of its associated sensations in your body, which may include feeling heaviness, sluggishness, fatigue, and tears.

On the flip side, if your emotion is happiness, how do you know happiness is there? Its associated feelings in your body may include smiling, wide-open eyes, tall posture, a hop in your step, being aware of your senses, and the feeling of being alive. And that all feels so amazing, right?

Take a moment to think of an emotion and how it makes you feel in your body. You can use the emotions listed above including anger, sadness, or happiness, or choose another. What did you learn?

YOUR 4 BEHAVIORS

It is stressful when an unwanted feeling or emotion is on board, and you may deal with it in 4 different ways. As I describe these 4 different behaviors, ask yourself, "Where do I see myself in these behaviors? What are my tendencies?" It could be one, more than one, or all of them. Here they are:

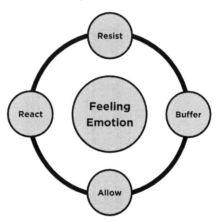

Do You RESIST?

Resisting is when you push away unwanted feelings and emotions. It's as if you are burying them under the ground, hoping they will just go away. But what happens when you do that? They grow even bigger and worsen, emerging even stronger later, which only perpetuates your undesirable feelings and emotions.

Do You REACT?

Reacting is when you quickly say something or do something that you really didn't mean to say or do. Usually you wish you could take it back. You may feel guilty after the fact, which can make you even more reactive.

Do You AVOID?

Avoiding is also known as buffering. It is when you use external behaviors to escape your unwanted feelings and emotions.

Do You ALLOW?

Allowing is simply *feeling* the feeling or emotion, even if it feels icky. This is the least commonly utilized choice even though it is the healthiest. We'll discuss this more later.

What did you discover about yourself in reviewing these 4 behaviors? What are your behavior tendencies?

MORE ON BUFFERING

> "If you don't know how to say no, your body will say it for you through physical illnesses."
>
> —Gabor Maté, M.D.

When you avoid or buffer, you choose a behavior in an effort to mask, cover up, or escape your unwanted feelings and emotions. Buffering creates distance between you and your feelings.

Buffering behaviors come in all shapes and sizes and can even include what may seem like healthy behaviors that become unhealthy when you overdo them. Doing too much of a good thing isn't healthy if it is done for the wrong reasons. What do I mean by that? For me, I used to buffer with exercise. I was an overexerciser, escaping my undesired emotions related to the stresses of burnout through too much fitness. Yes, too much fitness can be unhealthful when it causes wear and tear on your body, leading to injuries and pain, difficulty sleeping, exhaustion, doctor's visits, imaging studies, physical therapy, medications, and so on.

Here are some common ways people buffer:

- Alcohol
- Tobacco

- Vaping
- Misuse of prescription drugs
- Recreational drugs
- Gambling
- Overshopping
- Overeating and eating unhealthy foods
- Overexercising
- Frequent internet browsing
- Binge-watching TV
- Incessant cleaning or organizing
- Over-indulging in hobbies

Do you see yourself in any of these buffering behaviors? If so, which ones? Would you add any to the list?

BUFFERING IS A TEMPORARY FIX

Why does buffering feel so good? The answer is dopamine. Buffering releases dopamine, a "feel good" hormone. And when you feel good, you just want more and more of that feeling and therefore you continue the behavior. But keep this piece of wisdom in mind:

> "If you are trying to escape, you always have to be escaping. You can't get enough of something you don't really want."
>
> —Brooke Castillo, founder, The Life Coach School

Buffering doesn't produce positive outcomes. The good feeling is only temporary. And then you are left with the consequences of your actions that may have hurt you physically, emotionally, psychologically, and spiritually. Those consequences only lead to more negative thought loops, perpetuating your need to buffer.

THE ALCOHOL CULTURE

Many of my clients use alcohol as a buffer most frequently in the evenings after work and on the weekends. If you use alcohol to buffer, you are not alone. Alcohol is a particularly common buffer, and it's also a fairly dangerous one largely because of how culturally accepted it is.

I've never been a big drinker, but I grew up in a culture that normalized drinking when you're stressed and glamorized drinking in general. People were drinking in movies, magazines advertised cocktail recipes, and there was even an entire TV show that took place in a bar—*Cheers*.

Marketing and media portray alcohol as sexy and cool. And it's normalized to drink when you're upset. People often say, "I need a drink," when feeling stressed or they recommend a drink to others when they are feeling stressed.

That culture around alcohol hasn't changed. It's still everywhere. I live in an area that's very touristy and has a lot of microbreweries, and I see jokes about drinking printed on towels and home décor in stores. Many times, the first thing you're asked when you sit down in a restaurant is "Can I get you anything from the bar?"

Even though I've never been much of a drinker, there were times when I would come home stressed from work and would have a little sambuca or amaretto after dinner. I wasn't getting drunk, but I was reaching for alcohol. I liked the warmth. I liked how it calmed me down.

A Problem With My Drinking

A physician coach friend of mine, Dr. Kara Pepper, who openly shares about her relationship with alcohol, said something I thought was profound: "I didn't have a drinking problem. I had a problem with my drinking." That was exactly how I felt—I didn't have a problem in the sense that I was addicted to alcohol, requiring rehab. But the fact that I would reach for it every so often as a Band-Aid for how I was feeling, and that society taught me that was normal, was not okay. I didn't want alcohol to be an emotional crutch or a buffer for me.

Several decades ago, I stopped drinking completely. That change happened for 4 main reasons: First, I learned tools to relieve my stress to feel better all by myself, so I didn't need alcohol to calm me down anymore. Second, I noticed that I developed an intolerance to alcohol over time. Even if I had a bit of wine, I felt awful. I couldn't sleep, and I'd feel sluggish and dizzy the next day, lacking focus and concentration. Third, I didn't want to set a bad example for my children and have them thinking it was normal to reach for alcohol after a rough day. People frequently ask me, "Don't you miss it?" My answer is a flat-out no.

The fourth reason, and perhaps the most important, is that alcohol comes with some extremely detrimental health consequences.

WHY IS ALCOHOL A RISKY SUBSTANCE?

Not only did I feel awful when I consumed alcohol, but I learned that it's associated with and a direct cause of many illnesses and diseases. Being female and learning of alcohol's causal relationship with breast cancer was particularly alarming.

In his famous book *How Not to Die,* Dr. Michael Gregor wrote, "In 2010, the official World Health Organization body that assesses cancer risks formally upgraded its classification of alcohol to a definitive human breast carcinogen. In 2014, it clarified its position by stating that regarding breast cancer, no amount of alcohol is safe."

Among the general population, alcohol is responsible for a large number of problems, from negative health effects to accidents and even violence. According to the CDC, "Excessive alcohol use led to more than 140,000 deaths and 3.6 million years of potential life lost (YPLL) each year in the United States from 2015-2019, shortening the lives of those who died by an average of 26 years. Further, excessive drinking was responsible for 1 in 5 deaths among adults aged 20-49 years."

SHORT-TERM RISKS OF ALCOHOL USE

- Increases risk of injuries to self and others as a result of accidents (car crashes, drownings, burns, falls, etc.)
- Increases incidences of violence
- Can cause alcohol poisoning
- Increases risky sexual behaviors
- For pregnant women, can cause miscarriage, stillbirth, or fetal alcohol spectrum disorders (FASDs)

LONG-TERM RISKS OF ALCOHOL USE

- High blood pressure
- Heart disease
- Cerebrovascular accident (stroke)
- Liver disease
- Digestive problems

- Weakened immune system
- Dementia
- Learning and memory problems
- Depression
- Anxiety
- Alcohol use disorders or alcohol dependence
- Increased risk of several kinds of cancer:
  - Mouth and throat
  - Larynx (voice box)
  - Esophagus
  - Colon and rectum
  - Liver
  - Breast (in women)
  - Stomach
  - Pancreatic
  - Prostate

Many physicians struggle with alcoholism. Drinking among physicians in the U.S. has been increasing over time. In 2006-2010, 16.3% of physicians reported problematic alcohol use, which increased to 26.8% in 2017-2020.[62] This is particularly concerning because it's damaging not only to the health of physicians but also to their ability to care for patients.

Alcohol Is a Sensitive Subject

If you are buffering with alcohol, this may be a sensitive subject, and I know the thought of giving it up completely may be scary. But I am sharing this information because buffering with alcohol is very common and normalized and yet so very dangerous. I felt the need to lay out this information so you can make an informed decision. Just like I explained in the nutrition chapter—that I don't expect you to drop your current diet and become vegan—you don't have to completely quit all alcohol use immediately. Any change you make is better than no change. Focus on getting just 1% better every day. If you don't use alcohol as a buffer but are more of a connoisseur, occasionally pairing wine with food for example, you don't have to entirely quit something you enjoy. Your choice to drink alcohol is ultimately up to you.

CHOOSING TO ALLOW INSTEAD OF ESCAPE

When you want to escape a stressful, uncomfortable feeling or emotion, the first three behaviors I described—resisting, reacting, and avoiding/buffering—are all unhealthy behaviors with detrimental consequences. Not allowing yourself to feel your feelings and emotions causes "issues in your tissues," paving the way for illness.

Only one behavior in that list of 4 is actually healthy and that is *allowing*. Allowing is when you invite the unwanted feeling or emotion in for tea and conversation and listen to what it has to say. It's the key to understanding your thoughts. I know it will feel icky. I know it's unpleasant. I know you want to run the other way. But ask yourself this: "How successful have I been to date in getting through every unwanted feeling or emotion?" Do you know the answer? *It's 100%!* No matter how awful and stressful the feeling or emotion was, you have successfully made it through every time. So there is nothing to fear by inviting your feelings in and allowing them!

HOW TO ALLOW

> **Myth**: Saying no is just too hard.
> I need my buffers to get me through.
>
> **Truth**: Saying no is much easier when you utilize your stress relief tools so you don't need the buffers anymore.

If you don't allow your feelings and emotions, you may be wondering how to even begin. This is where your body-based and mindset stress-relief tools both come into play and work well when integrated together. Let me show you how.

TOOLS FOR ALLOWING

Part 1: Body-Based Tools

Unwanted feelings or emotions draw you to buffering behaviors (drinking, eating, buying, doing, etc.). I invite you to first try these body-based tools to help you process unwanted feelings and emotions prior to utilizing the mindset self-coaching tool. Remember it is more difficult to focus on your thoughts when your nervous system is dysregulated. Since you can't think a thought and feel a feeling in your body at the same time, it's best to start with bottom-up, body-based tools.

SHAKE IT OFF

1. Take off your socks and shoes and stand (if you are able) barefoot with your feet about hip distance apart.

2. Feel your feet touching the ground.

3. Either march in place or jump up and down for 20-30 seconds.

4. Pause for a moment and notice how you feel.

5. Shake your limbs one at a time, sensing the movements:
   - Left arm
   - Right arm
   - Left leg
   - Right leg

6. Shake opposite limbs, sensing the movements:
   - Left arm with right leg
   - Right arm with left leg

7. Pause for a moment and notice how you feel.

8. Fill out your worksheet for this tool. (StressFreeMD.net/worksheets)

9. If you enjoyed this tool, add it to your toolbox. (Page 35)

Shake It Off Video

5 SENSES MEDITATION

Your brain is receiving input from your 5 senses—touch, smell, taste, hearing, and seeing—at all times. But you are only consciously aware of about 10% of that input. The remaining 90% is subconscious. If you imagine an iceberg floating in the water, only the small portion that you can see above the water represents the senses that you are consciously aware of, while the rest of the iceberg represents the subconscious, under the water.

I like to think of your 5 senses as your "5 friends." Since you can't think a thought and feel a feeling at the same time, you can call on your 5 senses to help you emerge from your busy, thinking mind. This helps you come back into your body, which creates space in your mind to then work with the thoughts driving your feelings or emotions.

1. Find a comfortable seated or lying-down position. If you would like, remove your socks and shoes and if seated, feel your feet touching the ground.
2. Allow your eyes to soften or close.
3. Sense the parts of your body that are supported.
4. Sense the parts of your body that are lifted.
5. Sense your clothing touching your skin.
6. Sense the temperature of the air touching your skin that is not covered.
7. Notice any sounds inside your space or outside your space, and the sound of your own breath.

8. Notice any scents from your skin, hair, clothing, and the air surrounding you.
9. Notice any tastes in your mouth from the last thing you ate or drank.
10. Whether your eyes are open or closed, notice what you see: colors, shapes, shadows, textures, or light.
11. Sense your body breathing, lifting and lowering with each breath.
12. Pause for a moment and notice how you are feeling.
13. Fill out your worksheet for this tool. (StressFreeMD.net/worksheets)
14. If you enjoyed this tool, add it to your toolbox. (Page 35)

5 Senses Mediation Video

Part 2: Mindset Tool

After you have regulated your nervous system through your body-based tools and you feel calmer in your body, you are ready to work with your thoughts.

1. Get a piece of blank paper and a pen and record your answers.
2. From this place of calm, I invite you to *allow*—identify the unwanted feeling or emotion that drives you to buffer or escape, invite it in for tea and conversation, and listen to what it has to say.
3. Describe the main feeling or emotion.
4. Listen: What main thought is driving this feeling or emotion?
5. What situation drove that thought?
6. Notice how it was your thought about the situation, not the situation itself, that created your unwanted feeling or emotion and drove the buffering behavior.
7. What feeling or emotion would you like to have instead?
8. What thought better serves you and drives that desired feeling or emotion?
9. Think that thought. You can write it down on a sticky note or put it in the notes of your phone—someplace you have easy access.
10. Recognize how your buffering behavior is caused by your own thoughts that drive your unwanted feelings

and emotions, and when you allow those feelings or emotions from a place of calm, you no longer need the buffer.

11. Pause for a moment and notice how you're feeling.
12. Fill out your worksheet for this tool. (StressFreeMD.net/worksheets)
13. If you enjoyed this tool, add it to your toolbox. (Page 35)

Mindset Tool Video

PERMISSION TO TEMPORARILY COMPARTMENTALIZE

You may be thinking that you now understand that allowing yourself to feel your feelings and emotions is the truly the most healthy choice, but sometimes you are in a situation where you are not able to allow those feelings. In this case, I invite you to *temporarily* compartmentalize your unwanted feelings or emotions. Imagine putting them into a box and closing the lid with the understanding that you will open the lid and let them out when able.

It is common to have situations like that, and I've experienced it many times myself. I can think of a few memorable scenarios when this happened, both in and out of work. I remember being at my work desk reading out mammography cases when I received a call from my husband. I could tell immediately by his voice that something was wrong.

It was our son's first day at a new school in the 2nd grade, and it was the first time he was riding a school bus. My husband who was off of work that day went to the bus stop to pick him up after school. Our son did not get off the bus.

A few months prior, we'd taken a tour of the school with the principal and she'd asked if I had any concerns, and I specifically mentioned I was concerned about my son riding the school bus and getting lost. Now my fear had come to fruition. I was 45 minutes away from home with a ton of cases in front of me plus several scared patients I needed to see who were called back for additional diagnostic mammography and ultrasound imaging.

I could feel the heat and tension building in my body. I wanted to cry and scream. My mind was offering me terrifying thoughts about what could have happened to my son, and I wanted to just leave and find him. But I knew I couldn't leave. And I had to let my husband take care of it. In that moment, I needed to temporarily compartmentalize all of my feelings and emotions. It wasn't the place or time to allow them. Patients and staff depended on me and I needed to be there for them.

About an hour later, my husband called to tell me that my son was placed on the wrong school bus due to a typo on the teacher's roster and when he was the only student left on the bus, the bus driver followed protocol and brought him back to the school. It wasn't until after work when I got into my car in the parking lot that I was able to allow my feelings and emotions—predominantly fear about what could have happened, followed by gratitude for his safety.

So it is okay to temporarily compartmentalize as long as it's *only* temporary, with the understanding that you *will allow* your feelings and emotions when safely able. Repressed emotions cause stress and inflammation, tension, and elevated cortisol, which show up over time as illness.

Remember you have made it through 100% of every unwanted feeling and emotion that you have ever experienced. It may seem hard at first, but know that you are more than capable and you can do hard things.

> "If we all did the things we were capable of doing, we would literally astonish ourselves".
>
> —Thomas Edison

I invite you to astonish yourself!

* * * * * *

If you are in need, please seek help from a mental healthcare professional. Addiction is outside the scope of this book and should be treated by an addiction specialist. Addiction specialists deal specifically with this issue and can provide counseling and anti-relapse therapy.

* * * * * *

TIME TO TRANSFORM!

For a downloadable version of this worksheet, go to StressFreeMD.net/worksheets

BEHAVIOR CHANGE: ESCAPES

What behavior related to escapes would you like to change?

Identify your current stage in changing the behavior you identified above:

1. Precontemplation – *You don't believe that you need to change.*

2. Contemplation – *You're thinking about making a change within the next 6 months.*

3. Preparation – *You're aware of the need for change and plan on taking steps within 1 month. During this phase, you may set a goal and write out the steps you need to take.*

4. Action – *You've started making a change but have been doing it for less than 6 months and haven't yet reached your goal.*

5. Maintenance – *You've reached your goal and have sustained the desired behavior for more than 6 months.*

If you are not at least at stage 3, do the thought work necessary to get there. (Pages 38-42)

On a scale of 1-10, how confident are you that you can make the desired change?

        1 2 3 4 5 6 7 8 9 10

On a scale of 1-10, how important is it to you to make the change?

        1 2 3 4 5 6 7 8 9 10

If you scored lower than a 7 for either confidence or importance, do the thought work needed to score higher. (Pages 38-42)

If you scored a 7 or above, you're ready to set some goals.

CALMER GOALS

C: Clear – Be as clear and detailed as possible when describing what you want to achieve.

A: Assessable – You can assess if there has been any change in your behavior using concrete measurements.

L: Limited – Your goal has a limited time frame and scope, including a beginning and end date.

M: Meaningful – The goal is meaningful and applicable to your life and you understand why you want to achieve it.

E: Exciting – You feel excited to achieve your goal and know you can maintain motivation over an extended period of time.

R: Reachable – Your goal is not too much of an ask and is something you know you can really achieve.

What can you do to improve your stress with respect to escapes by just 1% today?

8

Stress Less, Thrive Better

"The secret of change is to focus all of your energy, not on fighting the old, but on building the new."

—Socrates

I'm cheering for you!

I'm Cheering for You Video

I'M CELEBRATING YOU!

You made it! Congratulations, and thank you for taking time for your amazing self. I know how busy you are and you could have been doing a gazillion other things, but you have instead prioritized yourself by focusing on your own well-being, and for this I celebrate you.

"If you don't make time for your wellness you will be forced to make time for your illness."

—Unknown

I know how overwhelming it can feel to try to reduce your stress alone, especially when you don't have the knowledge or the time to figure it out. Dr. Dean Ornish talks about replacing the "I" in illness with "we" to make "wellness." We are all in this together and I am grateful that you have chosen to spend your time here focused on your own wellness with me.

You and I = we!

NOW YOU CAN THRIVE, NOT JUST SURVIVE

What is the difference between thriving and surviving? I learned the distinction through my personal experience, and by witnessing my students on their cancer journey transform right before my eyes while I taught their weekly yoga therapy and meditation classes. At first, I saw them just surviving, coming into class with their heads down, quiet, making no eye contact, and shuffling to their mats. Then *boom*—a 180-degree shift, leaving class *fully thriving*, standing tall, socializing, making eye contact, and smiling with a skip in their steps, even asking for more frequent sessions. The term "cancer survivor" never sat well with me. I liked to call my students "cancer thrivers." Surviving is really about getting by, just barely living. But thriving means your life is fulfilled and you actually feel *alive*.

Thriving is how I feel now, and it's what I want for you. I hope you are beginning to feel like you can thrive rather than just survive after learning the what, why, and how of stress relief!

THE RIPPLE EFFECT

I wrote this book because I believe in my heart that everyone deserves to know what I know. It would feel selfish to keep all of my knowledge to myself. As the saying goes, "See one, do one, teach one," so I invite you to share what you have learned with others you care about, whether they are patients, colleagues, loved ones, or even someone angrily bagging your groceries at the market.

Studies show that physicians who practice the pillars of Lifestyle Medicine have a greater ability to motivate patients to change their behavior.[63] Physicians who take care of themselves are also more likely to educate their patients on healthy lifestyle choices.[64]

When I was a medical student, I remember seeing many healthcare professionals neglect their own health, and it sent a discordant message. One minute I'd be in the OR assisting my cardiothoracic surgery team in a quadruple bypass for extensive cardiovascular disease, and the next minute I'd be in the cafeteria watching those same surgeons eat cheesesteaks and drink sugary sodas. I thought, "Do they not remember what they just fixed? Do they think it couldn't happen to them?" Well, it did happen to at least one of my unhealthy surgery attending physicians.

Why would a patient listen to someone who isn't talking the talk and walking the walk?

If the patient sees their physician at the supermarket and their cart is full of fruits and veggies, it will make that patient think differently. If you embody healthy behaviors, your patients and the other people in your life are more likely to believe you, and you're more likely to talk about healthy behaviors with them.

> "The three most important ways to lead people are: by example, by example, by example."
>
> —Albert Schweitzer

Taking care of yourself not only elevates your own health but it elevates the health of others just by setting an example of what is possible. When people say to me "I want what she's having!" it validates that I am authentically living a healthful life.

STAY ORGANIZED

> "How you do anything is how you do everything."
>
> —T. Harv Eker

Our physician brains thrive best when organized. The key to your continued success in keeping your stress level low is to stay highly organized. So far I have helped to keep you organized through each chapter. Now I invite you to follow what works for me and my physician brain, which is to create a schedule.

Document your stress-relief tools in your daily schedule. It doesn't have to be anything fancy—I take a blank piece of paper and write everything I am doing with time slots, but you can choose something fancier like a Google sheet.

First off, I start my morning with meditation, yoga therapy, and exercise. This is the first thing I write down on my sheet. I write in when I can take breaks and what I will do on those breaks, such as getting outside and chatting with a friend. I include food prep and meals as well as sleep—yes, even sleep is included! Everything you do goes on that sheet. Once it's on the sheet, it becomes non-negotiable. Each entry is no different than a patient appointment. Think of your schedule as a series of personal appointments with yourself.

YOU ARE EXACTLY WHERE YOU NEED TO BE

> "Step aside from all thinking and there
> is nowhere you can't go."
>
> —Seng-Ts'an, third Founding Teacher of Zen

Now that you are feeling better, your brain may offer you some not-so-nice thoughts that fall into the "shoulda-coulda-wouldas," such as, "I should have known all of this already. I already wasted so much time and I could have felt better so much earlier in my life. If I only would have paid attention to my health sooner . . ."

The thing is, you don't know what you don't know. So drop the "what ifs" and focus on what *is*—where you are now. If you fall off the wagon of your self-care schedule, invite yourself gently back on. Nobody is perfect. I am not perfect. It happens. Know that whatever you do is more than doing nothing. It is enough. Remember you can improve exponentially by just growing 1% better each day.

> "We have two lives, and the second begins when
> we realize we only have one."
>
> —Confucius

Now go get it! It's yours for the taking.

Hungry for More?

> "Live as if you were to die tomorrow.
> Learn as if you were to live forever."
>
> —Mahatma Ghandi

Although my medical school interviews were several decades ago, there is one in particular that still stands out in my mind. While touring the gross anatomy lab at one medical school, I noticed this quote on the wall:

> "Knowledge is power."
>
> —Sir Francis Bacon

I love this! It is a reminder that you have the power in every moment to change the trajectory of your life. You have begun to do just that by spending quality time learning here with me through these chapters.

If you are like me, now that you have begun the process of implementing healthful stress-relieving behaviors, you are noticing how much better you feel! You may feel calmer, more grounded, and more rested. You may move with greater ease and feel less reactive. You may be more focused, with better concentration. Perhaps you've even become a kinder, gentler person to be around. You may notice that you are in need of fewer escapes. And, if you are like me, you have become hungry for even more! I am a lifelong learner and always seek out more of what makes me feel my best self.

This is not the end of your stress-relief journey—it is just the beginning! Now that this book has set your foundation, I invite you to learn about several additional ways to continue your stress-relief journey to elevate your lifespan and healthspan even further!

> "Education is not preparation for life.
> Education is life itself."
>
> —John Dewey

CONNECT WITH ME

How do you like to learn? Are you an auditory learner, a visual learner, or a tactile learner? Do you like to learn alone or with live individual or group support? No matter what your learning style is, I have created offerings that include all of these different ways of learning to best support you.

THE STRESSFREEMD PODCAST

Listen in for "stress-free snacks" from me as well as other experts. You can find hundreds of episodes streaming on your favorite platform as well as at https://podcast.stressfreemd.net/

HUNGRY FOR MORE?

PROGRAMS ON DEMAND

If you are someone who likes self-paced learning, check out these several programs on demand:

>https://www.stressfreemd.net/online-programs-on-demand

Rx Inner Peace: A Physician's Guide for Self-Care

This program combines online self-paced learning with 1:1 private coaching sessions:

>https://www.stressfreemd.net/rxinnerpeace

Self-Care Shop

Choose from six different online self-paced programs by topic:

>https://www.stressfreemd.net/selfcareshop

COACHING

1:1 Private Virtual Coaching

Personalized well-being programs designed to meet your specific well-being goals and desires for your flexible schedule:

>https://www.stressfreemd.net/1-1-coaching

REVIVE! LIFESTYLE MEDICINE WELL-BEING GROUP COACHING

Dive deeper into the pillars of Lifestyle Medicine combining both didactic and experiential learning in a group setting. This course can be tailored to meet the needs of your group by topics and time:

>https://www.stressfreemd.net/revive

SPEAKING

Looking for an interactive engaging speaker for your group, event or podcast? Inside or outside? Look no further. You found me! Contact me to discuss further:

> https://www.stressfreemd.net/speaker-presentations

RETREATS

Check out my upcoming retreats or invite me to create a retreat designed specifically for your group:

> https://www.stressfreemd.net/retreats

Once a cheerleader, always a cheerleader!
Cheering for you always!

Robyn

About the Author

Robyn Tiger, M.D., DipABLM, is a double board-certified physician in Diagnostic Radiology and Lifestyle Medicine. As founder of the wellness practice StressFreeMD, she uniquely combines her expertise in medicine, yoga therapy, meditation, and life coaching to teach other physicians a whole-person approach to relieve stress while increasing both lifespan and healthspan. Her innovative trauma informed courses, coaching, presentations, retreats, podcast, and book focus on creating effective behavior changes in the key topics of stress relief, nutrition, sleep, exercise, social connection, risky substances, and nature while cultivating physical, mental, and emotional well-being and resilience.

Robyn serves as lead faculty and subject matter expert in stress management for the *Foundations of Lifestyle Medicine Board Review Manual* and is a Western Carolina Medical Society Healthy Healer Partner.

Her journey into medicine began in the 3rd grade, when her teacher rolled out a life-sized human skeleton and she was beyond amazed. It was in that very moment that she knew she wanted to become a physician.

Robyn spent 15 years practicing Diagnostic Radiology, during which time she grew increasingly stressed, anxious, and sick with a host of mysterious symptoms that no specialist could diagnose. Just when she thought she'd run out of options, she attended a beginner yoga class and felt an unbelievable sense of calm. With a piqued curiosity, in an effort to help herself, she dove deeper into learning and applying more stress relief techniques. Over time, every last one of her mystifying symptoms vanished.

Beyond eager to learn the science behind what she'd experienced so she could share it with her fellow physicians, with whom she saw a particular need after having lost three of her colleagues to suicide, she became certified in yoga therapy, meditation, and life coaching. She eventually found her way to the American College of Lifestyle Medicine and was certified as a Lifestyle Medicine physician.

Her strong desire to help other physicians grew out of her own personal transformation following her many years in medical practice, experiencing firsthand the need for self-care education. She is deeply passionate about guiding others to become the best versions of themselves and live their healthiest, longest, and most fulfilling lives!

Resources

- **American College of Lifestyle Medicine**: LifestyleMedicine.org
- **International Association of Yoga Therapists**: iayt.org
- **iRest Institute**: iRest.org
- **The Life Coach School**: TheLifeCoachSchool.com
- **The Novato Institute for Somatic Research and Training**: SomaticsEd.com/novInstitute.html

Links

WORKSHEETS

All Worksheets
https://StressFreeMD.net/worksheets

VIDEOS

Welcome
https://vimeo.com/986152177/5dc25edbc8

How to Use This Book

Thought Work
https://vimeo.com/986146668/f8522e1c13

Behavior Change
https://vimeo.com/986148866/a3c9d8b3ab

Chapter 1

Cleansing Breath
https://vimeo.com/984594540/5f7705bc93

FEELING STRESSED IS OPTIONAL

Chapter 2

Straw Breath
https://vimeo.com/984602326/64d75725d5

Homunculus
https://vimeo.com/984609944/81c054744c

Cleansing Breath With Sound
https://vimeo.com/984619792/81289ffcf7

Straw Breath With Hug
https://vimeo.com/984622853/ab8bb9529e

Chapter 3

Mindful Eating
https://vimeo.com/986138503/65a054996e

Chapter 4

4-7-8 Breath
https://vimeo.com/984626144/4a30da0dfd

Guided Meditation for Sleep
https://vimeo.com/984630223/e178fbdc12

LINKS

Chapter 5

Progressive Muscle Relaxation
https://vimeo.com/984639744/0b39470c92

Posture Experiential
https://vimeo.com/984647804/4bb9653f91

Somatic Neck and Shoulder Release
https://vimeo.com/984650046/a089cd8f05

Chapter 6

The Power of Your Smile
https://vimeo.com/985337156/d65efe48eb

Loving Kindness Meditation
https://vimeo.com/985344035/a60c8d4d36

Chapter 7

What's Going Right?
https://vimeo.com/985360451/3ac01b4070

Shake It Off
https://vimeo.com/986131972/9d14b40743

FEELING STRESSED IS OPTIONAL

5 Senses Meditation
https://vimeo.com/985369615/c2303cfefd

Mindset Tool
https://vimeo.com/985377545/329ef8aef9

Chapter 8

I'm Cheering for You!
https://vimeo.com/986165431/5cbb5f51bf

Acknowledgments

"Piglet noticed that even though he had a very small heart, it could hold a rather large amount of gratitude."

—A.A. Milne

My comparatively small heart is immensely full with gratitude for so many amazing humans who have each played a vital role in the creation of *Feeling Stressed Is Optional*.

Oh, where to begin? I am teary as I write this. "Let's start at the very beginning, a very good place to start . . . " (Imagine Julie Andrews singing in *The Sound of Music*.)

To my oppressed ancestors who courageously left all that they had, speaking little to no English with not much more than the clothes on their backs, and emigrated to the U.S. in search of a better life. Not a day goes by that I am not eternally grateful that because of you, I get to live the life of your dreams. To my grandparents, who believed I could do anything. Your hearts beat on through me.

To all of my parents, Sandy, Henry, and Larry, beginning with my creation and entrance into this world to serve others and be the instrument by which they heal. Thank you for supporting me through the evolution of my unique journey in "doctoring others" in many different ways. To my mother-in-law, Bette, who calls me her "hero" and reminds me of my strength and purpose when I need it most.

To my father-in-law Mel's AIP—"Anything is possible." What I once thought was impossible became possible!

To my incredible husband, Eric, a.k.a. Prince Charming—". . . All of me loves all of you" (imagine John Legend singing)—for being my rock, always, and showing me daily how laughter is indeed wonderful medicine, and especially for your presence. To our incredible Tiger cubs, Benjamin and Elana, who have been my greatest teachers. Repeatedly seeing the world through your eyes has taught me to live with intention and release fear, reminding me of what is most important on life's journey. To our sweet pup Zoe, who sat at my feet while I studied for my many certifications and acted as my mock student while I practiced teaching my very first classes. To our adorable pup Yofi, who gives me unconditional love and oxytocin boosts daily to help me feel connected to others and to myself.

To my siblings, Ellyn and Richie, for cheering for me. I never get tired of hearing, "Go, Sis!" To Richie (yes, a second brother with the same name—we have a combined family), your cerebral palsy has placed you in the category of "special needs," but to me, this makes you just *special*. Your daily morning phone calls sharing your thoughts through the mind of a joyful child always bring a smile to my face, inviting me back to the present moment. To my in-law siblings, Michelle, Phil, Robert, and EV, for your caring support. To my nieces and nephews, Zac, Jake, Sam, Laynie, Dani, and Jack, for thinking I am a "cool aunt" and always being so interested in the "cool things" I am doing, raising my spirits and reminding me of my purpose.

To my dear friends who have lifted me, nourished me, shown me love and kindness, and been my mirror when I needed it most: Elyce Cardonick, M.D.; Beth Manin, M.D.; Nancy Roman, M.D.; Kim

ACKNOWLEDGMENTS

Senor; Brett Senor, M.D.; Nina Contino, MSS, CMSW; Melissa Sundermann, D.O.; Amy Comander, M.D.; Amber Orman, M.D.; Dawn Mussallem, D.O.; Christina Lucas Vougiouklakis, D.O.; Jonathan Fisher, M.D.; Brian Asbill, M.D.; Michelle Thompson, D.O.; Amy Vertrees, M.D.; Laurie Boge, D.O.; and Marci Falk.

To all of my brilliant educators: professors, teachers, instructors, attendings, mentors, coaches, and colleagues from so many different facets of my life, some still with us, others who have passed on, in the areas of medicine, yoga, yoga therapy, meditation, and coaching. Your teachings and trailblazing efforts are a composite of the person I have become.

From two of my mentors, I'd like to share meaningful words I cherish that have lifted me over the years:

"When someone asks you to do something don't say 'No, I don't know how.' Just confidently say 'Yes!' and then figure it out afterwards. You can do anything."

—Bernie Ostrum, M.D., Diagnostic Radiology

"Dear Robyn, a miracle is when everything (all factors) comes together just right for something special to happen. It's wonderful sometimes to watch how the amazing things come together for the amazing results. I think you are a miracle person."

—Eleanor Criswell, Ed.D., Founder Somatic Yoga, Novato Institute for Somatic Research and Training

Laurie Greene; Naida Burgess; Elaine Sherma; Joseph LePage; Lilian LePage; Maria Mendola Shamas; Genevieve Yellin; Karen O'Donnell Clarke; Debra Jensen; Tari Prinster; Camille Kittrell; Annie Okerlin; Molly Birkholm; Susan Pualani Alden; Karen Soltes; Robin Carnes;

Karen Lazarus; Shari Vilchez Blatt; Shanti Desai; Brenda Lyons; Pat Croce; Sunny Smith, M.D.; Hala Sabry, D.O.; Nneka Unachukwu, M.D.; Dena George, M.D.; Kate Mangona, M.D.; Brooke Castillo; Connie Mariano, M.D.; Miram Schwarz; Koushik Reddy, M.D.; Colin Zhu, D.O.; and Meagan Grega, M.D.

To Michael Greenfield for his warm welcome, trust, and support, giving me a home at Asheville Community Yoga to share my passion through in-person teaching offerings both East and West.

To Deepak Chopra, M.D., for his insightful guided meditations to begin my mornings with intention, potential, and focus. To Steve Brookner at the Ferguson YMCA and Peloton Interactive for keeping me strong in body and mind.

To my thousands of patients, clients, and students for entrusting your care and well-being education to me. Your enthusiasm in becoming your best selves is palpable and contagious in the best way possible!

To Laurie Johnson Photography for capturing my joy and passion.

To GreenCloud Apparel for the beautiful custom scrub attire worn in the videos.

To the amazing Aloha Publishing team: Maryanna Young, Megan Terry, Heather Goetter, Jen Regner, Nation Goetter, Mercy Sorich, Jodi Cowles Sherwood, Beth Berger, and Rachel Langaker. You said "Yes!" to my dream of many, many years and brought *Feeling Stressed Is Optional* to life. If it weren't for you, this would still be nothing but a dream. Your kindness, patience, insight, knowledge, creativity and inspiration fueled my passion and drive to completion. Because of you, together we are helping to elevate the health, well-being, and happiness of every human touched by this book. For this, I am forever grateful.

Book Club Questions

CHAPTER 1: PILLARS OF LIFESTYLE MEDICINE

What does living a healthy life mean to you? What motivations do you have to increase not just your lifespan, but your healthspan?

How are the pillars of Lifestyle Medicine prioritized in your life? What would you like to work on and why?

Did you learn something new or surprising from this chapter?

Did you learn anything you plan to share with others?

How did you feel when you tried your first stress relief tool? Did you find it helpful? Will you add it to your toolbox, and why? How could you incorporate it into your daily life?

CHAPTER 2: STRESS LESS, RELAX BETTER

How could your life improve by reducing the stress you experience on a daily basis?

What are the major stressors in your life? How many are related to work, health, and other external parts of life, and how many are psychological?

Stress is bidirectional. What factors of your life are affected by your stress, and how is stress affecting those areas of your life in return?

What did you feel when you tried the stress relief tools? What did you find helpful? What did you add to your toolbox and why? How could you incorporate these into your daily life?

Did you learn something new or surprising from this chapter?

Did you learn anything you plan to share with others?

CHAPTER 3: STRESS LESS, EAT BETTER

Have you noticed changes in your mood when you eat certain foods? If so, what foods affect you and how do you feel as a result?

What gets in your way of eating a healthier diet? What small changes can you make to your diet today to begin improving your eating habits overall?

Did you learn something new or surprising from this chapter?

What did you feel when you tried the stress relief tools? What did you find helpful? What did you add to your toolbox and why? How could you incorporate these into your daily life?

Did you learn anything you plan to share with others?

CHAPTER 4: STRESS LESS, SLEEP BETTER

Describe your typical attitude toward sleep. What do your current sleep habits look like? Did this chapter reveal anything to you about your quality of sleep?

What would an ideal sleep transition routine look like for you? Is there something you can do tonight to improve your sleep even a small amount?

What did you feel when you tried the stress relief tools? What did you find helpful? What did you add to your toolbox and why? How could you incorporate these into your daily life?

Did you learn something new or surprising from this chapter?

Did you learn anything you plan to share with others?

CHAPTER 5: STRESS LESS, MOVE BETTER

How much exercise do you currently get per week, and is that exercise mild, moderate, or vigorous?

What barriers get in your way of meeting the recommended exercise guidelines?

What type of exercise do you enjoy? Are you balanced in your exercise routine, including both cardiovascular and strength training?

How can you incorporate more movement in your daily routine?

What did you feel when you tried the stress relief tools? What did you find helpful? What did you add to your toolbox and why? How could you incorporate these into your daily life?

Did you learn something new or surprising from this chapter?

Did you learn anything you plan to share with others?

CHAPTER 6: STRESS LESS, CONNECT BETTER

Have you noticed feelings of isolation or loneliness in your life? If so, when?

Who of your acquaintances and friends can you reach out to and connect with intentionally, whether that's a text, phone call, a lunch date, or some other way?

How can you practice saying yes more often to social connections?

What did you feel when you tried the stress relief tools? What did you find helpful? What did you add to your toolbox and why? How could you incorporate these into your daily life?

Did you learn something new or surprising from this chapter?

Did you learn anything you plan to share with others?

CHAPTER 7: STRESS LESS, SAY "NO" BETTER

When faced with a negative feeling or emotion, do you tend to resist, react, avoid, or allow?

What kind of behaviors do you use to buffer your emotions? How can you create healthier behaviors that help you allow and process your feelings?

What did you feel when you tried the stress relief tools? What did you find helpful? What did you add to your toolbox and why? How could you incorporate these into your daily life?

Did you learn something new or surprising from this chapter?

Did you learn anything you plan to share with others?

CHAPTER 8: STRESS LESS, THRIVE BETTER

What has been your overall experience in reading the content and learning the tools in this book?

How can living with less stress improve your life and the lives of those around you?

Which tools have you accumulated in your toolbox? Are there any tools you regularly practice now? What has been most helpful for you and why?

Have you shared anything you've learned throughout this book with others?

What was your favorite quotation throughout this book?

What steps are you planning to take next to reduce your stress and live a happier, healthier life? What can you do to improve by just 1% today?

Podcast and Media Questions

1. How has learning stress relief techniques changed your life?
2. Why is it important for physicians to learn effective stress relief methods?
3. How does managing stress improve health outcomes?
4. What got you started on your journey to become board certified in Lifestyle Medicine?
5. What makes Lifestyle Medicine different from other approaches to medicine?
6. What compelled you to write this book?
7. What was the most rewarding experience throughout your book writing journey?
8. What is the one stress relief technique you wish everyone would practice daily?
9. What makes your book unique from other wellness and stress management books?

Citations

1. *Physician Lifestyle and Happiness Report 2023*, Medscape 2023, https://www.medscape.com/sites/public/lifestyle/2023

2. Nerurkar, A., et al. When physicians counsel about stress: results of a national study. *JAMA Intern. Med.* 2013; 173(1):76-77. doi:10.1001/2013.jamainternmed.480

3. Bodell, Lisa. 2022. New Year's resolutions fail. Do this instead. *Forbes*, Dec. 19. December. https://www.forbes.com/sites/lisabodell/2022/12/19/new-years-resolutions-fail-do-this-instead/

4. Ornish, D., Scherwitz, L.W., and Billings, J.H., et al. Intensive lifestyle changes for reversal of coronary heart disease [published correction appears in *JAMA* 1999 Apr 21;281(15):1380]. *JAMA*. 1998;280(23):2001-2007. doi:10.1001/jama.280.23.2001

5. Woolf, S.H., et al., Life expectancy and mortality rates in the United States, 1959-2017. *JAMA*. (2019) 322:1996-2016.

6. Seaward, B.L. *Managing Stress: Principles and Strategies for Health and Well-Being*, 8th edition. Jones & Bartlett Learning. 2014.

7. Nerurkar, A., et al., When physicians counsel about stress: results of a national study. *JAMA Intern. Med.* 2013; 173(1):76-77. doi:10.1001/2013.jamainternmed.480

8. McCall, T. *Yoga as Medicine*. Bantam Books. 2007.

9. Ornish, D., Lin, J., and Daubenmier. J., et al. Increased telomerase activity and comprehensive lifestyle changes: a pilot study [published correction appears in *Lancet Oncol*. 2008 Dec; 9(12):1124]. *Lancet Oncol*. 2008; 9(11):1048-1057. doi:10.1016/S1470-2045(08)70234-1

10. Kane, Leslie, M.A., "I Cry but No One Cares" *Physician Burnout & Depression Report 2023*, Medscape 2023, https://www.medscape.com/slideshow/2023-lifestyle-burnout-6016058?icd=login_success_gg_match_norm

11. "What is physician burnout?" *American Medical Association*, February 16, 2023. https://www.ama-assn.org/practice-management/physician-health/what-physician-burnout

12. Office of the U.S. Surgeon General. "Addressing Health Worker Burnout: The U.S. Surgeon General's Advisory on Building a Thriving Health Workforce" *U.S. Department of Health and Human Services* 2022. https://www.hhs.gov/surgeongeneral/priorities/health-worker-burnout/index.html

13. Wessinger, Dave. 2023. Clinician Burnout Goes Beyond Staffing Shortages—How Technology Can help. *Forbes*, Jan. 17, 2023. https://www.forbes.com/councils/forbesbusinesscouncil/2023/01/17/clinician-burnout-goes-beyond-staffing-shortages-how-technology-can-help/

14. Brazeau, C.M., Shanafelt, T., Durning, S.J., Massie, F.S., Eacker, A., Moutier, C., Satele, D.V., Sloan, J.A., and Dyrbye, L.N. "Distress among matriculating medical students relative to the general population." *Acad Med.* 2014 Nov; 89(11):1520-5. doi: 10.1097/ACM.0000000000000482. PMID: 25250752

15. Ishak, W., Nikravesh, R., Lederer, S., Perry, R., Ogunyemi, D., and Bernstein, C. "Burnout in medical students: a systematic review." *Clin. Teach.* 2013 Aug; 10(4):242-5. doi: 10.1111/tct.12014. PMID: 23834570.

16. 2020 AAMC Association of American Medical Colleges: https://www.aamc.org/

17. Dyrbye, L.N., Massie, F.S. Jr., Eacker, A., et al. "Relationship between burnout and professional conduct and attitudes among US medical students." *JAMA*. 2010; 304(11):1173-1180. doi:10.1001/jama.2010.1318

18. Guille, C., Zhao, Z., Krystal, J., Nichols, B., Brady, K., and Sen, S. "Web-Based Cognitive Behavioral Therapy Intervention for the Prevention of Suicidal Ideation in Medical Interns. A Randomized Clinical Trial." *JAMA Psychiatry*. 2015; 72(12):1192–1198 Academic Medicine: July 2017 - Volume 92 - Issue 7 - p 976-983; doi: 10.1097/ACM.0000000000001736

19. Kane, Leslie, M.A., "I Cry but No One Cares" *Physician Burnout & Depression Report 2023*, Medscape 2023, https://www.medscape.com/slideshow/2023-lifestyle-burnout-6016058?icd=login_success_gg_match_norm

20. Edwards, S.D., Edwards, D.J., and Honeycutt, R. "HeartMath as an Integrative, Personal, Social, and Global Healthcare System." *Healthcare (Basel)*. 2022; 10(2):376. Published 2022 Feb 15. doi:10.3390/healthcare10020376

21. Murray, C.J., Atkinson, C., Bhalla, K., et al. The state of US health, 1990-2010: burden of diseases, injuries, and risk factors. *JAMA*. 2013; 310(6):591-608. doi:10.1001/jama.2013.13805

22. Cleveland Clinic. "Americans Concerned About Their Weight, but Don't Understand Link to Heart Conditions and Overall Health." Cleveland Clinic Newsroom. January 31, 2019. https://newsroom.clevelandclinic.org/2019/01/31/americans-concerned-about-their-weight-but-dont-understand-link-to-heart-conditions-and-overall-health

23. *Physician Lifestyle and Happiness Report 2023*, Medscape 2023, https://www.medscape.com/sites/public/lifestyle/2023

24. Chen, M., Li, Y., Sun, Q., et al. Dairy fat and risk of cardiovascular disease in 3 cohorts of US adults. *Am. J. Clin. Nutr.* 2016; 104(5):1209-1217. doi:10.3945/ajcn.116.134460

25. Sarris, J., Logan, A.C., Akbaraly, T.N., et al. Nutritional medicine as mainstream in psychiatry. *Lancet Psychiatry*. 2015; 2(3):271-274. doi:10.1016/S2215-0366(14)00051-0

26. Li, Y., Lv, M.R., Wei, Y.J., et al. Dietary patterns and depression risk: A meta-analysis. *Psychiatry Res.* 2017; 253:373-382. doi:10.1016/j.psychres.2017.04.020; Jacka, F.N., Pasco, J.A., Mykletun, A., et al. Association of Western and traditional diets with depression and anxiety in women. *Am. J. Psychiatry*. 2010; 167(3):305-311. doi:10.1176/appi.ajp.2009.09060881; Jacka, F.N., Pasco, J.A., Mykletun, A., et al. Association of Western and traditional diets with depression and anxiety in women. *Am. J. Psychiatry*. 2010; 167(3):305-311. doi:10.1176/appi.ajp.2009.09060881

27. McGill, C.R., Fulgoni, V.L., 3rd, and Devareddy, L. Ten-year trends in fiber and whole grain intakes and food sources for the United States population: National Health and Nutrition Examination Survey 2001-2010. *Nutrients.* 2015; 7(2):1119-1130. Published 2015 Feb 9. doi:10.3390/nu7021119

28. de Vos, W.M., Tilg, H., Van Hul, M., and Cani, P.D. Gut microbiome and health: mechanistic insights. *Gut* 2022; 71(5):1020-1032. doi:10.1136/gutjnl-2021-326789

29. Li, Y., Lv, M.R., Wei, Y.J., et al. Dietary patterns and depression risk: A meta-analysis. *Psychiatry Res.* 2017; 253:373-382. doi:10.1016/j.psychres.2017.04.020

30. Beezhold, B.L., and Johnston, C.S. Restriction of meat, fish, and poultry in omnivores improves mood: a pilot randomized controlled trial. *Nutr. J.* 2012; 11:9. Published 2012 Feb 14. doi:10.1186/1475-2891-11-9

31. Conner, T.S., Brookie, K.L., Richardson, A.C., and Polak, M.A. On carrots and curiosity: eating fruit and vegetables is associated with greater flourishing in daily life. *Br. J. Health Psychol.* 2015; 20(2):413-427. doi:10.1111/bjhp.12113; Beezhold, B., Radnitz, C., Rinne, A., and DiMatteo, J. Vegans report less stress and anxiety than omnivores. *Nutr. Neurosci.* 2015; 18(7):289-296. doi:10.1179/1476830514Y.0000000164

32. Ornish, D., Magbanua, M.J., Weidner, G., et al. Changes in prostate gene expression in men undergoing an intensive nutrition and lifestyle intervention. *Proc. Natl. Acad. Sci. USA.* 2008; 105(24):8369-8374. doi:10.1073/pnas.0803080105

33. Ornish, D., Madison, C., Kivipelto, M., et al. Effects of intensive lifestyle changes on the progression of mild cognitive impairment or early dementia due to Alzheimer's disease: a randomized, controlled clinical trial. *Alzheimers Res. Ther.* 2024; 16(1):122. Published 2024 Jun 7. doi:10.1186/s13195-024-01482-z

34. Ornish, D., Scherwitz, L.W., Billings, J.H., et al. Intensive lifestyle changes for reversal of coronary heart disease [published correction appears in *JAMA* 1999 Apr 21; 281(15):1380]. *JAMA.* 1998; 280(23):2001-2007. doi:10.1001/jama.280.23.2001

35. Okello, E., Omagino, J., Fourie, J.M., Scholtze, W., Nel, G., Scarlatescu, O., and Lwabi, P. 2020. *Uganda Country Report*. PubMed Central (PMC) (1. August). doi:10.5830/CVJA-2020-037, https://doi.org/10.5830/CVJA-2020-037.

36. Jenkins, D.J., Kendall, C.W., Marchie, A., et al. Effects of a dietary portfolio of cholesterol-lowering foods vs. lovastatin on serum lipids and C-reactive protein. *JAMA*. 2003; 290(4):502-510. doi:10.1001/jama.290.4.502

37. Zhang, Y., Zhuang, P., Wu, F., et al. Cooking oil/fat consumption and deaths from cardiometabolic diseases and other causes: prospective analysis of 521,120 individuals. *BMC Med*. 2021; 19(1):92. Published 2021 Apr 15. doi:10.1186/s12916-021-01961-2

38. Czeiser, C.A. Medical and genetic differences in the adverse impact of sleep loss on performance: ethical considerations for the medical profession. *Transactions of the American Clinical and Climatological Association* 2009; 120:249.

39. Pacheco, D., and Rehman, A., M.D. 2023. Drowsy Driving vs. Drunk Driving: How Similar Are They? *Sleep Foundation*. 3 November. https://www.sleepfoundation.org/drowsy-driving/drowsy-driving-vs-drunk-driving

40. Powell, N.B., Schechtman, K.B., Riley, R.W., Li, K., Troell, R., and Guilleminault, C. The road to danger: the comparative risks of driving while sleepy. *The Laryngoscope* 2001; 111(5):887-893.

41. Rimer, J., Dwan, K., Lawlor, D.A., et al. Exercise for depression. *Cochrane Database Syst. Rev.* 2012; 11(7):CD004366. Published 2012 Jul 11. doi:10.1002/14651858.CD004366.pub5

42. Fishman, L.M. Yoga and Bone Health. *Orthop. Nurs.* 2021; 40(3):169-179. doi:10.1097/NOR.0000000000000757; Lu, Y.H., Rosner, B., Chang, G., and Fishman, L.M. Twelve-Minute Daily Yoga Regimen Reverses Osteoporotic Bone Loss. *Top. Geriatr. Rehabil.* 2016; 32(2):81-87. doi:10.1097/TGR.0000000000000085

43. Griffin, É.W., Mullally, S., Foley, C., Warmington, S.A., O'Mara, S.M., and Kelly, Á.M. Aerobic exercise improves hippocampal function and increases BDNF in the serum of young adult males. *Physiology & Behavior* 2011; 104(5):934-941.

44. Moore, S.C., Patel, A.V., Matthews, C.E., et al. Leisure time physical activity of moderate to vigorous intensity and mortality: a large pooled cohort analysis. *PLoS Med.* 2012; 9(11):e1001335. doi:10.1371/journal.pmed.1001335

45. Aya, V., Flórez, A., Perez, L., and Ramírez, J.D. Association between physical activity and changes in intestinal microbiota composition: A systematic review. *PLoS One* 2021; 16(2):e0247039. Published 2021 Feb 25. doi:10.1371/journal.pone.0247039

46. *Physician Lifestyle & Happiness Report 2024*, Medscape 2024, https://www.medscape.com/sites/public/lifestyle/2024

47. U.S. Department of Health and Human Services, President's Council on Sports, Fitness & Nutrition, Facts and Statistics: physical activity. https://health.gov/our-work/nutrition-physical-activity/presidents-council#footnote-3

48. Strain, T., Flaxman, S., Guthold, R., Semenova, E., Cowan, M., Riley, L.M., Bull, F.C., Stevens, G.A., and the Country Data Author Group. National, regional, and global trends in insufficient physical activity among adults from 2000 to 2022: a pooled analysis of 507 population-based surveys with 5.7 million participants. *Lancet* June 25, 2024. https://www.thelancet.com/journals/langlo/article/PIIS2214-109X(24)00150-5/fulltext

49. van der Ploeg, H.P., Chey, T., Korda, R.J., Banks, E., and Bauman, A. Sitting time and all-cause mortality risk in 222 497 Australian adults. *Arch. Intern. Med.* 2012; 172(6):494-500. doi:10.1001/archinternmed.2011.2174

50. Matthews, C.E., George, S.M., Moore, S.C., et al. Amount of time spent in sedentary behaviors and cause-specific mortality in U.S. adults. *Am. J. Clin. Nutr.* 2012; 95(2):437-445. doi:10.3945/ajcn.111.019620

51. Dunstan, D., Barr, E., Healy, G., et al. Television viewing time and mortality: the Australian diabetes, obesity and lifestyle study (AusDiab). *Circulation* 2010; 121(3):384.

52. Kesaniemi, Y.A., Danforth, E., Jensen, M.D., Kopelman, P.G., Lefèbvre, P., and Reeder, B.A. Dose-response issues concerning physical activity and health: an evidence-based symposium. *Medicine & Science in Sports & Exercise* 2001; 33(6):S351-S358.

CITATIONS

53. Wen, C.P., Wai, J.P., Tsai, M.K., et al. Minimum amount of physical activity for reduced mortality and extended life expectancy: a prospective cohort study. *Lancet* 2011; 378(9798):1244-1253. doi:10.1016/S0140-6736(11)60749-6

54. Hennenlotter, A., Dresel, C., Castrop, F., Ceballos-Baumann, A.O., Wohlschläger, A.M., and Haslinger, B. The link between facial feedback and neural activity within central circuitries of emotion—new insights from botulinum toxin-induced denervation of frown muscles [published correction appears in *Cereb. Cortex* 2010 Jan; 20(1):253. Baumann, Andres O. Ceballos [corrected to Ceballos-Baumann, Andres O.]]. *Cereb. Cortex* 2009; 19(3):537-542. doi:10.1093/cercor/bhn104

55. One smile can make you feel a million dollars. *The Scotsman*. https://www.scotsman.com/health/one-smile-can-make-you-feel-a-million-dollars-2469850

56. Eisenberger, N.I. The neural bases of social pain: evidence for shared representations with physical pain. *Psychosom. Med.* 2012; 74(2):126-135. doi:10.1097/PSY.0b013e3182464dd1

57. Grant, W.T. Study of Adult Development. *Harvard Second Generation Study*. 2015.

58. Office of the Surgeon General. 2024. Social connection. HHS.gov. 15. July. https://www.hhs.gov/surgeongeneral/priorities/connection/index.html

59. Kannan, V.D., Veazie, P.J. 2023. US trends in social isolation, social engagement, and companionship - nationally and by age, sex, race/ethnicity, family income, and work hours, 2003–2020. SSM, *Population Health* 21 (1. March): 101331. doi:10.1016/j.ssmph.2022.101331, https://www.ncbi.nlm.nih.gov/pmc/articles/PMC9811250/

60. Kannan, V.D., and Veazie, P.J. U.S. trends in social isolation, social engagement, and companionship - nationally and by age, sex, race/ethnicity, family income, and work hours, 2003–2020. *SSM Popul. Health* 2023; 21:101331. https://www.ncbi.nlm.nih.gov/pmc/articles/PMC9811250/

61. *Physician Lifestyle and Happiness Report 2023*, Medscape 2023, https://www.medscape.com/sites/public/lifestyle/2023

62. Brooks, M. 2022. Problematic alcohol use on the rise among physicians? Medscape, 21. December. https://www.medscape.com/viewarticle/985957?form=fpf

63. Oberg, E., and Frank, E. Physicians' health practices strongly influence patient health practices. *The journal of the Royal College of Physicians of Edinburgh.* 2009; 39(4):290.

64. Abramson, S., Stein, J., Schaufele, M., Frates, E., and Rogan, S. Personal exercise habits and counseling practices of primary care physicians: a national survey. *Clinical Journal of Sport Medicine* 2000; 10(1):40-48.

Made in United States
Troutdale, OR
11/24/2024

24684148R00135